Healthy Back Basics

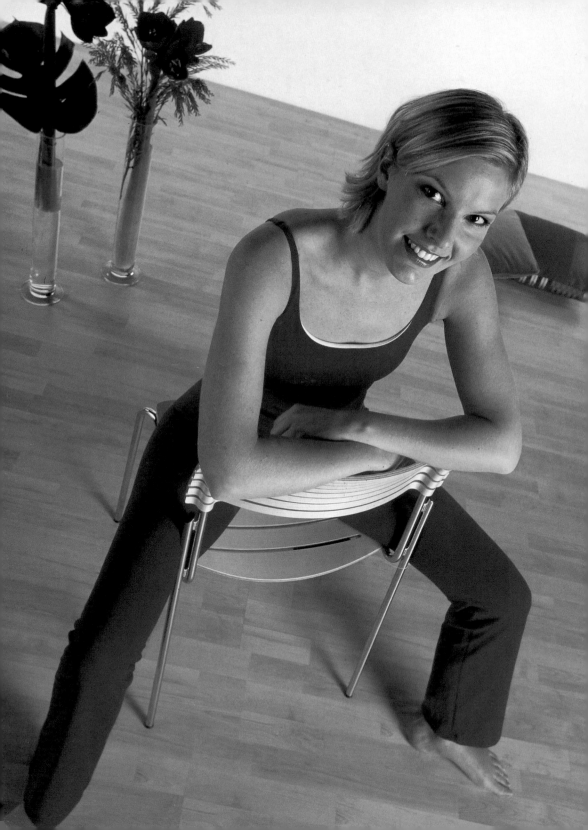

Healthy Back Basics

Helmut Reichardt

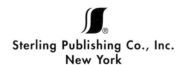

Sterling Publishing Co., Inc.
New York

Translated from the German by Anne Jahn

Library of Congress Cataloging-in-Publication Data Available

10   9   8   7   6   5   4   3   2   1

Published by Sterling Publishing Co., Inc.
387 Park Avenue South, New York, NY 10016
Originally published in Germany under the title *Rückenschule*
für jeden Tag by BLV Verlagsgesellschaft mbH, München
Copyright © 2004 by BLV Verlagsgesellschaft mbH, München
English Translation Copyright © 2006 by Sterling Publishing Co., Inc.
Distributed in Canada by Sterling Publishing
$^{c}/o$ Canadian Manda Group, 165 Dufferin Street,
Toronto, Ontario, Canada M6K 3H6
Distributed in the United Kingdom by GMC Distribution Services,
Castle Place, 166 High Street, Lewes, East Sussex, England BN7 1XU
Distributed in Australia by Capricorn Link (Australia) Pty Ltd.
P.O. Box 704, Windsor, NSW 2756, Australia

Manufactured in China
All Rights Reserved

Sterling ISBN-13: 978-1-4027-3098-6
        ISBN-10: 1-4027-3098-5

For information about custom editions, special sales, premium and corporate
purchases, please contact Sterling Special Sales Department at 800-805-5489 or
specialsales@sterlingpub.com.

Contents

Why Should You Do Back Exercises?

Few health questions receive as much attention as that of whether or not to do back exercises. In the last few years many books have been published that deal with back exercises, and you may wonder what makes this one different. For one thing, *Healthy Back Basics* is exercise-focused, although we do provide brief explanations of the theoretical foundations behind certain exercises when necessary. We believe that if you understand *why* you are exercising, you will be more motivated to adhere to a regimen. However, we will not delve too deeply into why a specific technique works, because we want to replace theory with action. Once you have experienced the health benefits of these exercises, you will know how to keep your back healthy and strong for a long time to come.

What kind of exercises are these?

The exercises we describe are calisthenics, which means you do not need any equipment to perform them. We have made them simple, so you can follow them without further instruction and do them anytime and anywhere. Our exercises target the entire body and are offered as general suggestions.

■ Only you and your doctor can determine which exercises are appropriate for you. Always consult a professional if you have special concerns or a history of back problems.

This book is not intended to point out your "faults." Don't exercise simply because you want to avoid a guilty conscience! Try the exercises and figure out which ones actually make you feel better by helping to improve your posture and habitual body movements.

In order to successfully exercise your back, you must pay

attention to your body. This book is meant to encourage you to change your habits by becoming more active and changing your everyday behavior. It shows simple exercises you can easily understand and perform. You do not need any materials other than your body and common household objects. Take it easy with the exercises, give yourself time and space to experiment, and enjoy yourself.

Find out how good it feels to have a strong back!

What is body awareness, anyway?

Body awareness means, simply, becoming more familiar with your body. You have to live with it your entire life. This may sound amusing, but it should also make you think about how you view your own body—what you know about it and how you treat it. Again, because *Healthy Back Basics* is an exercise-focused book, this will not be discussed in depth. However, you should start thinking about your body perception and how it relates to your posture.

Listen to your body.

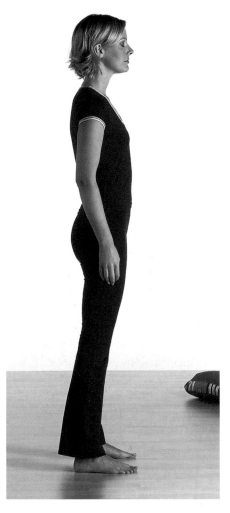

Exercise is more than a replacement for physical activity, which tends to be minimal in our sedentary society.

Exercise does not just improve your physical condition.

It is also a key element in keeping in touch with your body. That's why it's important for you to concentrate while exercising: Consciously controlling your musculoskeletal system provides access to your body. Pay attention to how you feel throughout the exercises and how your body reacts to them.

■ EXAMPLE

Stand up straight with your feet hip-width apart, keeping your arms relaxed. Shift your weight forward while you lift your heels off the ground until you are balancing on the balls of your feet. Focus on a point on the ground in front of you. Close your eyes after making sure that you can maintain your balance in this position. Open your eyes after a couple of seconds and return to the starting position with your feet flat on the ground. This easy exercise is one way to become aware of your body.

Life is movement; thus, improving your habits of movement will contribute to the quality of your life.

Think about that statement: Being alive does not mean simply functioning biologically; it also means being active.

Over the course of your life, you develop individual patterns of posture and movement. Parallel to the history of your life is the history of the way in which your body has moved. Statements such as "he looks beat" or "has the weight of the world on his shoulders" reflect some of the ways we *physically* respond to life and its responsibilities.

You may also say someone "jumps for joy" or "has her chin up" to express the connection between a person's posture and state of mind. How you feel affects how you look—and vice versa.

Although the effects of endurance training have been widely studied, there is scant research dealing specifically with the relationship between posture and mental condition. Yet the benefits associated with good posture and exercise—including decreased susceptibility to stress and increased general well-being—cannot be ignored.

The connections we make between movement and body awareness are based on empirical data gained from practices that have been shown to help bring about a positive inner transformation and an improvement in one's attitude.

■ EXAMPLE

Stand upright with your feet hip-width apart. Raise your heels off the ground while slowly shifting your weight forward until you are balancing on the balls of your feet. Keep your eyes open. Remain in this position for a few seconds, then go back to standing flat on your feet comfortably again. Step forward with one foot while making sure that the toes of both your feet point straight ahead. Shift your weight to the front leg, then press the heel of the back foot down toward the ground. Simultaneously straighten the knee of the back leg until you feel your calf muscles stretch.

■ Relax after a couple of seconds and go back to standing on the balls of your feet. Do you notice any difference in how your legs feel? The one you have just stretched may feel warmer or more relaxed.

We encourage you to pay attention to your posture and the habits affecting it, and exercise is a great way to start that process. As you become more conscious of your body you will take more responsibility for it, which will in turn increase your

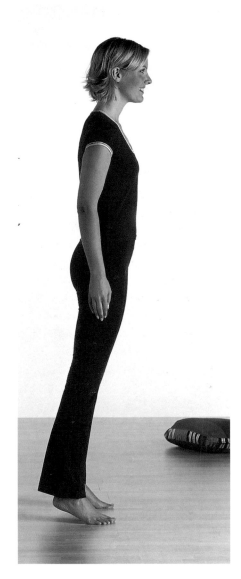

Feel your body.

well-being.

This book shows you how to behave more sensibly in everyday situations and how to perform appropriate exercises for improving your physical condition. You should "move" more sensibly as soon as you get up in the morning and remain attentive to this throughout your day.

The exercises we present are simple, easy to follow, and designed to help improve your habits and patterns of movement. They do not require a typical gym setting and can be easily incorporated into your routine, allowing you to be active while doing your daily tasks and wearing your regular clothes. You will begin to notice common sequences of movements as well as your postural habits.

You need not exercise at specific times or for long periods to improve your physical condition. With our plan, *you* determine which exercises you find helpful—as well as when to do them. If you are not a "morning person," for example, you probably won't be enthusiastic about exercising right after waking up. Finding a time of day that is comfortable and convenient for you will increase your chances of success.

Relax when you exercise. Do not force yourself. Rather, try to enjoy working out. Perform the different exercises several times to discover which ones work for you. Then begin to incorporate them into your day. Even small changes to your posture or the way you sit can make a big difference in how you feel.

Seeing an improvement in your physical condition will not only motivate you to stay in shape but may help you spot— and change—other negative habits. If you agree that "life is movement; thus, improving your habits of movement will contribute to the quality of your life," you have here an excellent opportunity to get to know your body—which, after all, has to last you a lifetime.

Is a straight back really straight?

Human evolution is linked to the development of an upright posture. The human body, especially the skeletal system, had to undergo many changes to facilitate a bipedal, or two-legged, lifestyle. Most notably, the spine transformed into the central axis of a bipedal skeletal structure on account of the different effect that gravity had on it compared with the earlier, four-legged stage. In response to gravity, the human spine evolved from the single curve of a four-legged creature to a double-S shape, which absorbs shocks and other strains.

The typical human spine is almost exactly in line with a person's center of gravity. This allows for efficient use of the muscles involved in maintaining balance. There is an obvious relationship between your posture and the muscles that you use, a relationship that is also a major focus of this book.

The spine adapts to the strain it has to endure. The cervical (neck-level) spine is

Be conscious of your posture and movement.

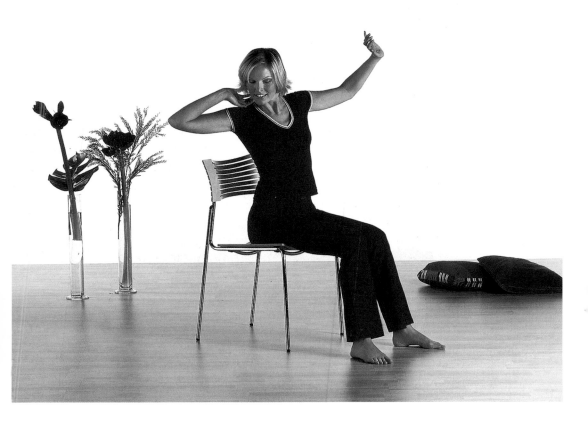

relatively stable, while the lower parts of the spine consist of massive vertebrae and sections of great mobility. The spine is curved in the area that connects the pelvis to the lumbar vertebrae. The vertebrae in this area have adjusted to the shape of the spine so that their surfaces are aligned parallel to one another, which maintains an even balance of stress on the intervertebral disks. The lumbar spine is particularly susceptible to strain, and can be damaged by assuming and holding positions that alter the curve of the spine.

One major cause of lumbar damage is our sedentary lifestyle: Modern humans spend most of the day sitting—at work, in school, or at home. While it's true that you can purchase a chair that will provide additional support and cushioning to accommodate the natural curve of the lumbar spine, you should work toward actively using your muscles to support your spine instead of relying on a backrest. Failure to make use of your muscu-loskeletal system regularly will weaken your muscles. For that reason, many of the exercises in this book target the lumbar spine.

■ **The curvature of the spine helps it to absorb shocks and strains.**

Questions and Answers

Does sitting bend my back?

Many chairs are shaped like the one pictured here. The woman is sitting in a typical way. We will explain the structure of the human spine in more detail so that you understand what happens when you sit down.

As humans evolved toward an upright posture, our lumbar spine naturally curved forward (toward the stomach), as you can see in the photo on the following page. Our individual vertebrae are shaped and positioned in such a way that their surfaces are parallel when we are standing upright. In this position there is equal strain on each of the disks located between the vertebrae. When you change your position from standing to sitting, you bend your hip joints while tilting your pelvis forward. This causes the lumbar spine to move in the opposite direction and the vertebrae to put more pressure on the anterior sections of the disks, both of which contribute to back pain. Furthermore, the abdominal and back muscles tend to be relaxed when you sit, resulting in even less support for the spine.

Consider the more deliberate

Hunching your back while sitting strains your intervertebral disks.

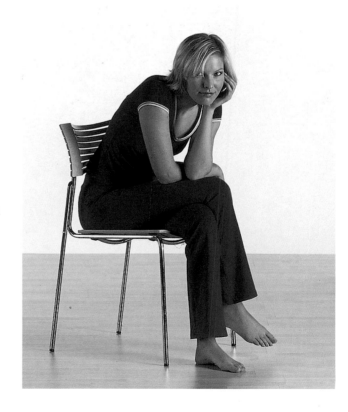

seated posture pictured below. Sit in the front half of your chair. Set your feet hip-width apart so that your buttocks and your knees form a triangle. Arch your back and tilt your pelvis backward until you are sitting on your gluteal muscles. Now tilt your pelvis forward while simultaneously straightening your back until you feel your hip bones. Imagine that your head is being pulled upward by a string, like a

puppet. Your lumbar spine is now in a position similar to the one you are in when standing upright. Feel the different positions of your pelvis by touching your hips.

Sitting in the way we just described improves the distribution of strain on the intervertebral disks and is therefore better for your back. You will find it more tiring than your accustomed posture because it actively uses your muscles. Do not go back to a slumped position. Give yourself time to let your back muscles gradually adapt to supporting your spine. Eventually abandon the backrest in favor of active muscular support that will decrease the stress on your skeletal system.

Do not just imitate the exercises by assuming the poses you see in the photos; try to *feel* how tilting your pelvis affects your lumbar spine and how to straighten your cervical spine. Then adopt only the habits of sitting that you experience as helpful and comfortable. Long-term success is determined primarily by your personal sense of well-being.

Sitting up straight relieves the strain on intervertebral disks.

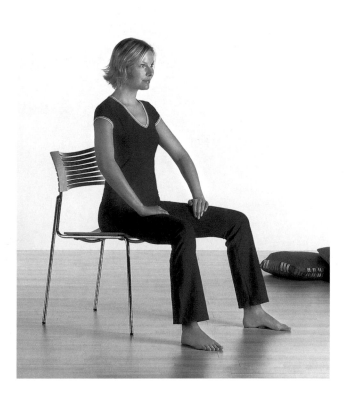

■ **TIP:**

Tilting your pelvis while you sit makes it easier to straighten your spine and decreases strain on the intervertebral disks.

Active sitting is something you have to learn.

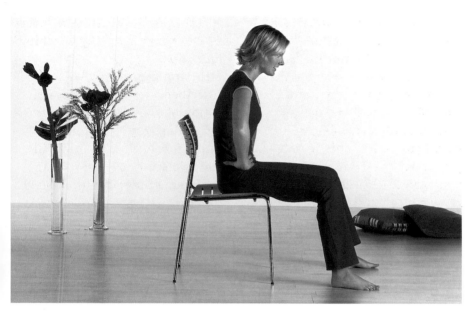

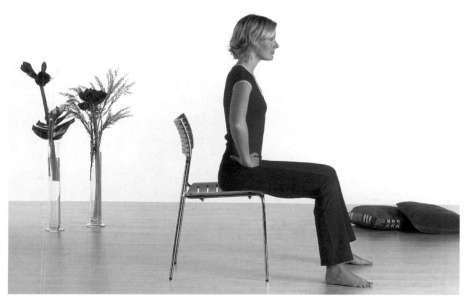

Are ergonomic chairs better for my back?

Pictured here is a typical ergonomic chair. The seat tilts forward and there is no backrest. Such a chair can help angle the pelvis, which promotes a healthy spinal position, but you cannot just sit in an ergonomic chair and expect to see improvement—you must learn how to use it correctly. If your back muscles are to replace a backrest, they must develop the strength to do so. They will need time to adjust to this role, so be sure to actively practice sitting in the chair, taking regular breaks.

Because an ergonomic chair does not guarantee a sitting position that respects the curve of your spine, it is always

Tilting your pelvis a little bit will facilitate sitting up straight.

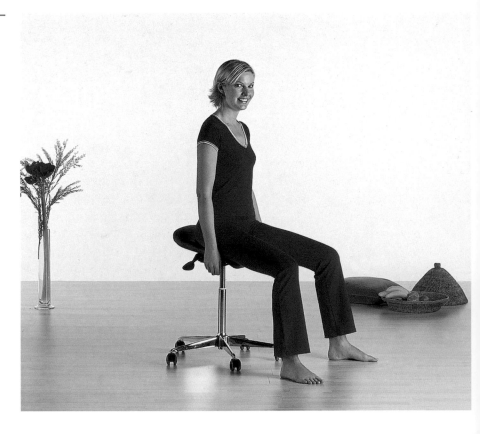

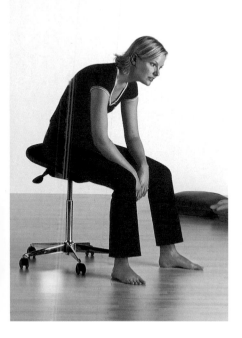

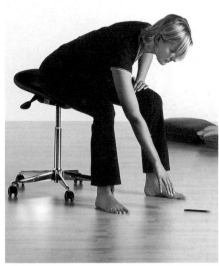

important to hold your muscles effectively when sitting upright. If you relax them, you will start to slump.

When you choose a chair, make sure the angle and the height of its seat are adjustable. Buy a chair that rotates to allow the greatest possible mobility. And don't forget to think about your style of dress when making your selection; for example, it is almost impossible to sit on an ergonomic chair in a tight skirt or high heels! Therefore, it's not enough simply to buy any chair with a tilted seat. You should consider the position of your spine and experiment sitting in the chair the same way you experiment with exercise.

As previously mentioned, the backward curve of the spine puts a great deal of strain on the skeletal system, and thus also on the intervertebral disks. Even with both feet flat on the ground you must actively use the muscles of your torso.

When you relax these muscles, your spine returns to a slumped position. When you lean over, make sure that your feet touch the ground so that you lower your upper body, flexing your hip muscles. In the example pictured, the woman is lowering her upper body within her natural range of movement. We will further explain this in the following section.

Taking a "relaxed-sitting" break aids in resting your back.

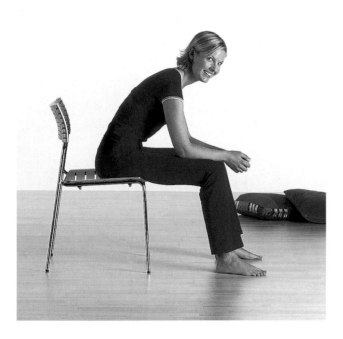

How do I sit on conventional chairs?

We've explained how most chairs force you to sit in a position that is bad for the spine. The musculoskeletal system is usually able to compensate for this as long as you are sufficiently active. However, if you have a job in which you spend most of the time sitting, or if you already suffer from a spinal disorder, you should pay more attention to the way you sit.

The following exercises show sitting positions in which the spine is supported by its surrounding muscles. We will show you how to minimize strain on your musculoskeletal system in common situations.

Keep in mind what we said earlier about sitting in such a way that allows the spine to curve naturally. Sitting with a stable spine is the starting position for the following exercises. Let your muscles adjust gradually to new activities by taking plenty of short breaks. You can also give your muscles a rest by stretching regularly.

■ REMINDER:

When you sit in the front half of the chair, set your feet firmly on the ground, about hip-width apart. Tilt your pelvis so that your lumbar spine assumes its natural, curved shape. Straighten your thoracic (chest-level) spine. This requires you to use your back muscles actively.

Keep your legs in the starting position as pictured on page 18. Do not rely on the back of the chair to support your spine. Place your forearms on your thighs while you sit up straight. Slowly arch your back while using your arms for support. Your upper body is now balanced and you no longer need to support it with muscular tension. If this "relaxing" position is uncomfortable for you, however, take a break by standing up for a moment.

Tilting your pelvis is crucial for keeping the lumbar spine in a healthy position. Adjusting the angle of your chair can help you arrive at the right stance. You can use a wedge-shaped foam pillow to achieve the proper angle when sitting in a conventional chair. Make sure that your seat tilts slightly forward. It is important that you straighten your thoracic spine, even when you use such a pillow.

Once you are able to support this position with the muscles of your torso—while you work at your desk, for example—start paying attention to other habits that affect your spine.

Sit with your legs slightly more than hip-width apart so that your thighs and your knees form an equilateral triangle. You should always maintain this angle with your thighs.

A wedge-shaped pillow can facilitate good posture.

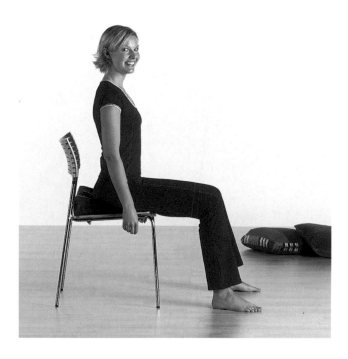

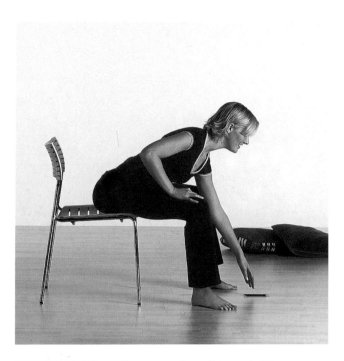

Paying attention to the angle of your back will relieve strain on your spine.

good for your spine. For example, you can use the back of your chair to support your arms (although you may not be able to do this at work). If you do have the opportunity to turn your chair around, take advantage of it. The chair back forces you to spread your legs. This stabilizes the lumbar spine. Support your torso by placing your forearms on the back of the chair. In addition, the position of your arms should help you straighten your thoracic spine.

How do I strengthen and stretch my back?

When you bend to get files or pick up an object from the floor, observe the angle formed by your thighs. Maintain the contraction of your torso muscles and lower your upper body at the hip joint to decrease strain on the spine.

Because it is not performed within the triangle formed by your thighs and knees, bending sideways as shown in the left-hand photo on page 21 causes your spine to twist, putting considerably more strain on it.

There are different techniques for sitting in a position that is

The musculature of the human body has evolved in order to adapt to an upright posture. Certain muscle groups have undergone changes that are similar to those that occurred in the skeletal system. Some muscle groups with motor functions in tetrapods (four-legged vertebrates) began to take on support functions in bipeds (two-legged vertebrates). Other muscle groups with support functions in tetrapods took on motor functions in bipeds. Although the affected muscle groups have

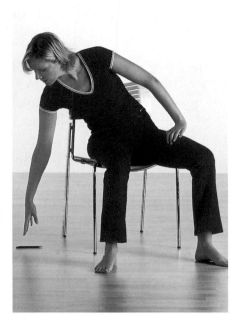

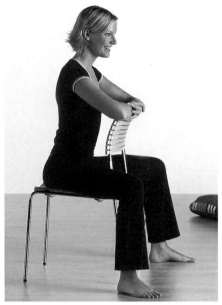

Disregarding the proper angle of your back while bending will strain your spine.

Supporting your forearms will relieve your pectoral spine.

adapted to their new functions, some still have features that are suited to their former function, with muscles previously controlling motor functions being less tense than other supporting muscles and vice versa. This is crucial information in physical therapy because it explains why certain groups of muscles tire more easily than others. This also explains why some muscles are more flexible than others.

■ **You should strengthen and stretch your muscles for best results.**

Which muscles should I stretch?

The Pectoral Muscles

The large muscles of your chest move your arms forward and turn them inward. Stretch them by moving your arms toward

Pectorals

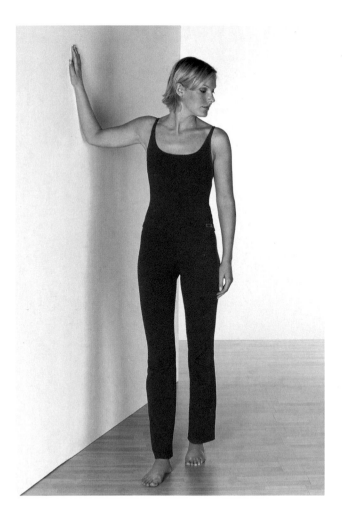

your back and twisting them outward as far as possible.

The Hip Flexors

The iliac muscles are composed of your loin muscle, which originates in the lumbar spine, and a muscle coming from the pelvic basin. These are the strongest flexing muscles of the hip joint. Straightening the joint—taking care not to tilt your pelvis or lumbar spine—will stretch the muscles.

Although they are part of the hip flexors, the quadricep muscles do not have a large effect on the hip joint. Their main function is to straighten the knee joint and can be stretched only by straightening your hip while bending your knees. You will distinctly feel these muscles as you stretch them.

The Muscles of the Inner Thigh

The adductor muscles of the thigh close your legs. Stretch them by moving your legs outward. This group of muscles is composed of many individual muscles with different functions. Keep that in mind while you stretch your hips by bending at

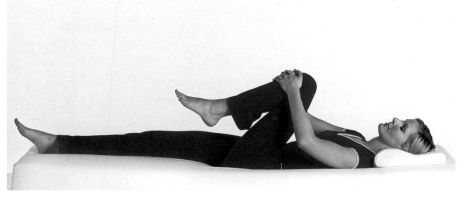

Hip flexors

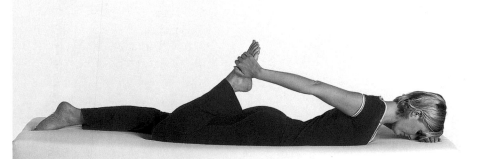

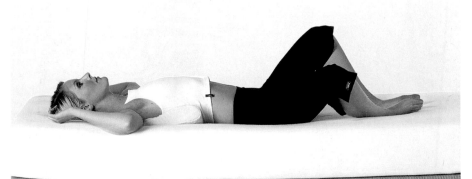

The inner-thigh
muscles

different angles. If you keep your pelvis stable, you can also stretch each leg separately.

The Neck Muscles

The upper parts of the trapezius have stabilizing as well as motor functions. They support and carry the shoulder girdle and move the head. When contracted on one side, these muscles simultaneously turn the head and tilt it sideways. You can stretch them by slowly cocking your head to each side.

The Shoulder Muscles

The levator scapulae muscles stabilize the shoulder girdle and allow you to raise your shoulders. They also support the cervical spine. Contracting these muscles on one side causes your head to turn and tilt to that side. Stretch them by tilting and turning your head in the opposite direction.

Pain or tension around the shoulder blades is usually caused by these muscles.

Neck and
shoulder muscles

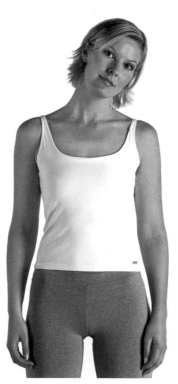
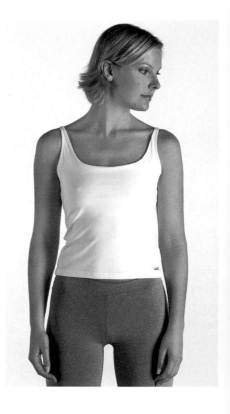

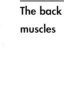

The back
muscles

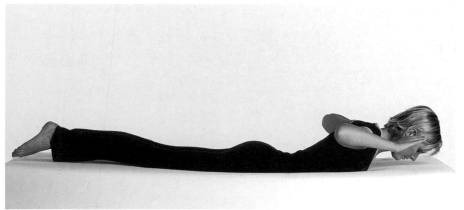

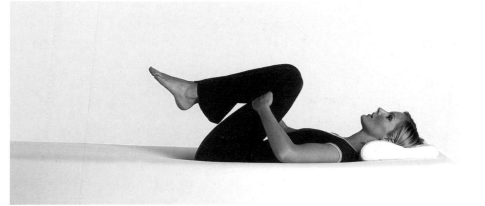

The Back Muscles

The extensor muscles of the back are a complex functioning unit that supports and stabilizes your body. The back muscles need to be kept flexible because they also perform many motor functions and tend to be less flexible than most muscles with motor functions. The back extensors are commonly underdeveloped. For this reason, we provide exercises that strengthen as well as stretch them.

The Hamstring Muscles

Above:
Hamstring
muscles

Below: Calf
muscles

The back of your thigh is made up of strong individual muscles. These muscles affect the joints in your hips and knees. They have both motor and support functions. You must know the motor function of a muscle in order to stretch it. Always stretch a muscle in the direction opposite to its habitual movement.

Stretch your hamstring by bending your hip joint and then straightening your knee joint. *The order is important!* Always bend your hips first and *then* straighten your knees.

The Calf Muscles

The calf muscles are made up of two muscles lying on top of each other. The outer section consists of a "two-headed" muscle—one that attaches in two distinct places on the same side—and a deeper muscle that is one-headed. The deeper muscle originates in the back of the lower leg; the two-headed originates in your thigh, slightly above the knee joint. Both of these muscles end at the Achilles tendon, which is connected to the heel bone. Stretch your calf muscles by straightening your knee joint while tilting your foot up toward the knee.

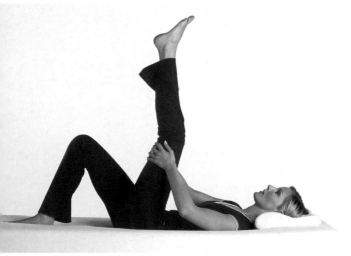

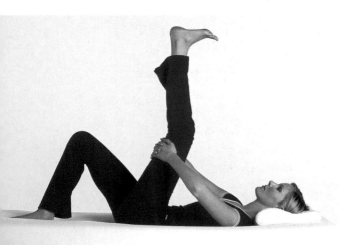

What's the best way to stretch?

The skeletal muscles can contract, but they also have elastic properties that can be developed. When the musculoskeletal system is not active enough, especially due to sedentary or bad postural habits, the muscles adjust by becoming stiff and less flexible.

Concentrate on the muscle group you are stretching. Pay attention to how your muscles feel when you stretch and when you relax. Hold the stretching position for several moments, then release. Avoid quickly switching back and forth between stretching and relaxing. If you are already used to doing stretching exercises, you can try to contract your muscles prior to stretching.

■ Wearing high heels over long periods of time can cause the calf muscles to constrict, diminishing their flexibility. If you wear high heels, never begin exercising without warming up! You could damage your muscles or Achilles tendon. Lifting the heel tilts the pelvis, which causes swayback.

Imagine you are pushing against an object. Build up tension and maintain it for about five seconds. Then stretch the muscle in the opposite direction. You should not overcontract your muscles; moderate contraction is enough preparation for stretching.

Hold the position for about ten seconds while exhaling. Once you are more advanced, you can determine your own stretching intervals.

Which muscles should I strengthen?

Lower-Leg Muscles

The muscles in your calf lift the outer edges of your foot. Your anterior shin muscles raise your instep. Strengthen both muscle groups with specific foot exercises (see top photo on page 28).

The Shoulder Girdle

The lower sections of the trapezius muscle draw your shoulder blades down toward your spine. These muscles support your shoulder blades and stabilize your shoulder

Leg muscles

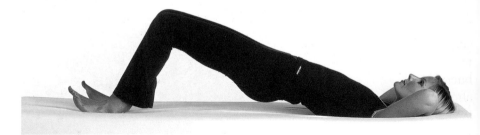

girdle during movement at or above shoulder level.

The rhomboideus muscle group, located to the left and right of your spine, draws your shoulder blades inward. These muscles stabilize the shoulder girdle.

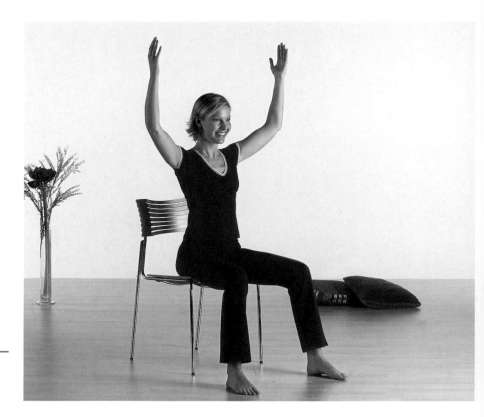

The muscles of
the shoulder
girdle

The Shoulder-Blade Muscles

The anterior coracoid muscles, located at the side of the rib cage below the chest muscles, move your arms forward and backward. They stabilize the shoulder girdle during various types of movement. Together with the rhomboideus muscles mentioned before, they form a sling that supports the shoulder blades (see left-hand photo on page 30).

The Gluteal Muscles

The intermediate and small gluteal muscles spread your legs apart from your hip joints.

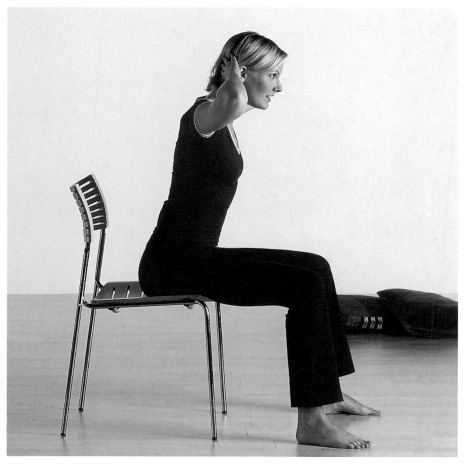

Muscles of the shoulder girdle

Shoulder-blade muscles

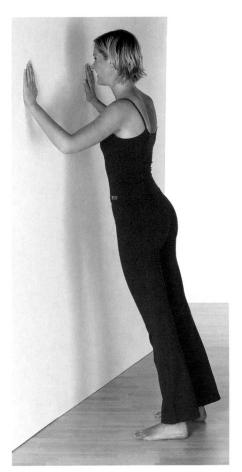

These muscles support the pelvis and, therefore, the spine. Strong gluteal muscles are crucial for upright posture (see lower photo on page 31).

The Hip Muscles

The large gluteal muscles straighten your hip joints. However, if the hip flexors are not flexible enough, the gluteal muscles do not reach their functional potential. This can be addressed by effectively combining strengthening exercises with stretching (see top picture on page 31).

The Abdominal Muscles

Your abdominal muscles consist of multiple parts that function together. The main abdominal muscles connect the rib cage to the pelvis, flex the torso, and

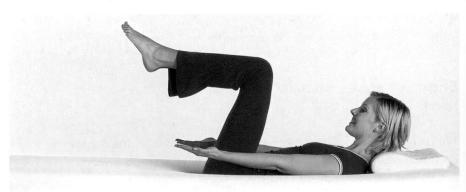

Abdominals

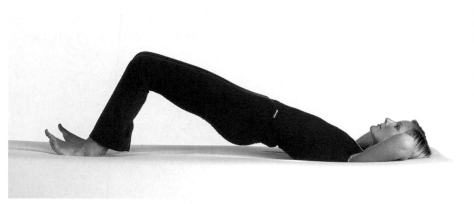

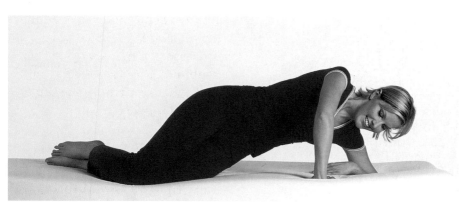

Above: Hip
flexor muscles

Below: Pelvis-
stabilizing
muscles

support the trunk. The oblique abdominal muscles flex and turn your upper body and support the spine.

Should I build muscle or focus on posture?

We provide several exercises to help improve posture. You can actively contract your skeletal muscles by sending nerve impulses, which stimulate them. A nerve impulse is an electrical stimulus that originates in nerve cells within the spinal marrow. These cells are connected to the brain, which gives the "order" for your muscles to contract. A single nerve cell coordinates the multiple muscle fibers of skeletal muscles.

A nerve cell and its corresponding muscle fibers are called a motor unit. While many motor units contract when exposed to strong stimuli, significantly fewer respond to weak stimuli. The potential strength of individual muscles depends on the overall number of muscle fibers and the capacity to activate those fibers at the same time, both of which can be developed through exercise. Exercise trains the fibers of individual muscles to work together more smoothly while improving the coordination among muscle groups.

■ **Develop muscle coordination by exercising regularly.**

The muscles that make up your musculoskeletal system are connected to the cerebrum, which controls voluntary movement and allows you to contract and relax your muscles at will. Note that your brain does not "decide" to use individual muscles; it always "imagines" complete postures and movements, storing their patterns within the cerebral cortex. This gives you the ability to automatically perform familiar sequences of movements in a well-coordinated way without focusing on them. It takes time to internalize new patterns before you can coordinate your muscles just as naturally. The same applies to postural habits and to movements that have to be relearned.

■ **Your brain needs time to store changes of postural habits and movement.**

Your musculoskeletal system sends many signals to the brain through specialized sensors able to detect different stimuli. That's how you know that you are feeling something press against your skin or that your muscles are tense. Once these signals reach the brain, they are processed and a return message is sent to the musculoskeletal system. All of this takes place unconsciously; however, you can observe these processes by focusing on your movement. Practice this by trying to imagine at what angle your arm is bent without looking at it.

Body awareness helps you understand the connection between your posture and the way you move.

How your body reacts to exercise is very individual. For example, some people describe their muscles as feeling warm or heavy after stretching.

■ **Becoming conscious of your body will bring information to the surface that normally escapes your attention.**

Keeping your muscles active affects your musculoskeletal system in many ways:

- Muscular activity stimulates the cerebral cortex. After multiple muscle contractions, even of different muscle groups, a person generally feels stimulated. You unconsciously do just that when you stretch after waking up.
- Muscular activity also stimulates your breathing activity.
- Blood circulation in muscles increases during the relaxation phase following activity. This is often experienced as a warm or "burning" sensation in the muscles that have just been exercised.
- It is easier to relax your muscles after they have contracted. You can take advantage of this by contracting and then stretching a muscle before you exercise it.
- Static muscle tension activates your circulatory system. This may affect you negatively if you do not breathe freely while you exercise.
- The tension in your muscles will increase. This helps muscles that have a naturally diminished tension. Your muscles also gain strength from being exposed to strong stimuli.
- Over a longer period of time you will see your patterns of posture and movement improve. Focus on adopting new patterns until your brain remembers them and performs them naturally.

The list above demonstrates that the effect of the cerebrum on your musculoskeletal system is not a simple matter of cause and effect, as there is also a reaction from the muscles that acts on the brain.

The Cervical Spine: Mobility and Stability

We have already spoken a bit about the difference between bipeds, vertebrates that walk on two legs, and tetrapods, which walk on four. Another, critical, difference is in the way the skull and its joints attach to the spine; this is what allows a human being's head to balance upright on top of the cervical spine, as opposed to the head of the tetrapod, which hangs down.

Pain or disability in the cervical spine is very common in humans and is often caused by weak or chronically relaxed muscles. Strengthening and stretching exercises that target this area of the cervical spine are recommended. You will notice that some of the exercises in this book require an unusual sequence of movements. This helps illustrate the basic function of individual muscle groups.

Many people cannot completely straighten their cervical spine. These exercises will help you to do so. Stand up straight in front of a mirror. Look forward and focus on a single point. Now tilt your head back slowly. Keep your gaze on the same point in the mirror and make sure your shoulders stay relaxed throughout the exercise.

Stand up straight again, tilting your head forward this time. Make sure to keep your head at the same level. Do not move your shoulders or upper body.

Repeat this a few times, then do the following to stretch your neck muscles: Imagine that you are being pulled upward by a thread, like a puppet. Repeat the movements in this position with a straightened cervical spine.

If you have difficulty relaxing your shoulders, hunch them upward, as in the left-hand photo on page 36. Keep your head centered and be sure not to tilt it backward. Slacken and lower your shoulders. Your shoulders should feel warm while relaxing.

■ TIP:
Do not move your cervical spine without stabilizing it with your muscles.

Although many of these exercises are presented in a standing position, you can also do most of them while sitting. It's especially important to do them whenever you are sitting for extended periods of time.

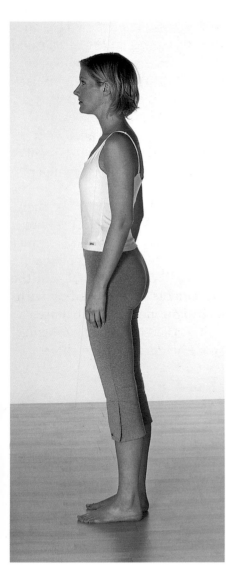 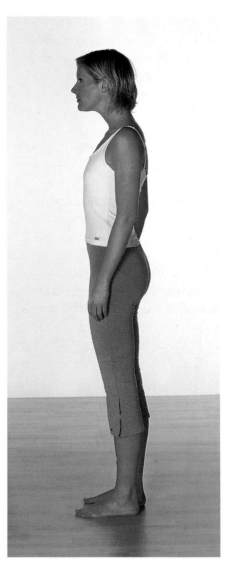

Mobilizing the cervical spine

■ TIP:

Relax your neck and shoulders by raising your entire shoulder girdle while keeping your arms relaxed.

The next exercises are done in front of the bathroom mirror: Roll up a towel and, grasping both ends, place it behind your neck. Pull the ends of the towel forward while you push against it with your neck. Straighten your cervical spine by using the towel to raise your head toward the ceiling.

Watch yourself in the mirror.

Stabilizing the cervical spine

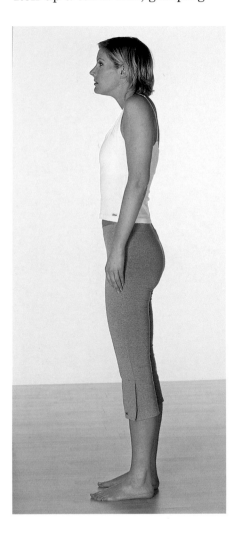
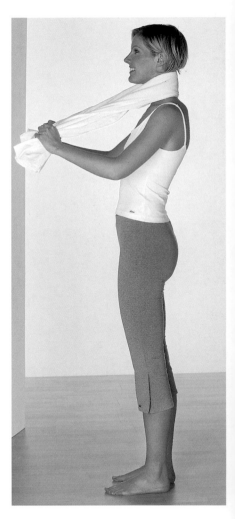

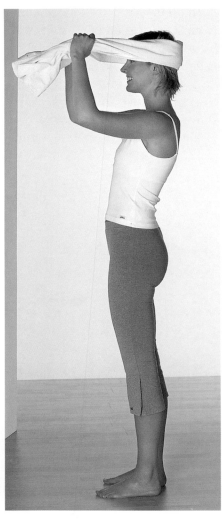
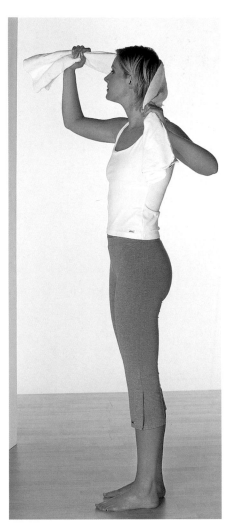

Slowly build up the intensity of the muscular contraction. Make sure to breathe freely during the exercise. Never hold your breath.

You can also perform this exercise by placing the towel against the back of your head, as shown in the left-hand photo above. Be careful not to let the towel slip during the exercise. Raise your head toward the ceiling while increasing tension in the muscles.

Always mobilize
the cervical spine
slowly and
without forcing it.

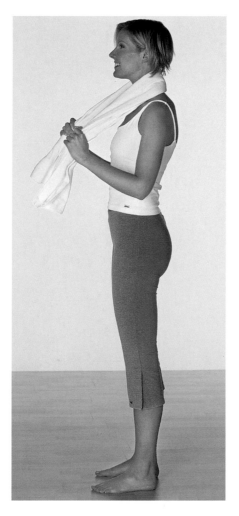

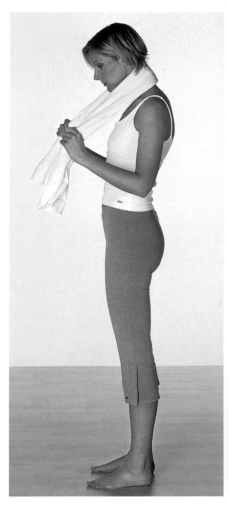

Keeping the towel in the same position as in the previous exercise, pull one end forward while pushing against it with your head, as shown in the right-hand photo on page 37. Do not build up the contraction too much, as it may cause your head to slip from the towel. Breathe freely throughout the exercise.

In the next exercise, stand up straight with the towel at the nape of your neck. Pull both ends forward and bend your head down until your chin reaches your rib cage.

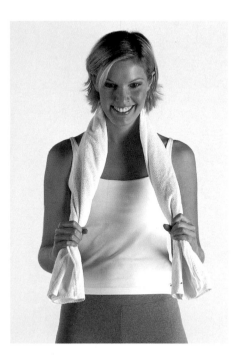

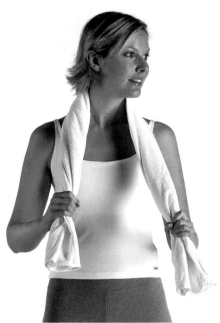

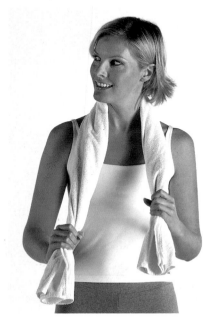

Keeping your upper body stable, slowly pull your head back up. Do not follow the movement of your head with your upper body.

Place the towel at the nape of your neck again and gently pull the ends forward. Bend your head slightly, looking down at the floor. Turn your head to the side without changing the position of your cervical spine and maintain the contraction for a couple of seconds. Slowly release the tension and repeat on the other side.

For the next exercise, hold

the towel in the same position. Keep your head centered between your shoulders. Pull the ends of the towel forward while pushing against it with your neck. Turn your head to either side while maintaining the contraction. Breathe freely throughout the exercise.

The following exercise has the same starting position. Again pull the towel forward while pushing your neck against it. Now tilt your head to either side. Look at yourself in the mirror to check the position of your head and neck.

You can also do these exercises without a towel while sitting in your office or during your lunch break.

The exercise on page 41 targets the upper section of the cervical spine.

Turn your head to the side. Lower your eyes and look at your shoulder. Let your head follow your gaze. Then look toward the ceiling. Again, let your head follow your line of sight.

The upper part of the cervical spine is again mobilized, this

More variations

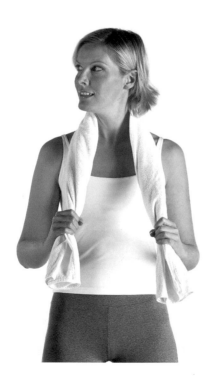
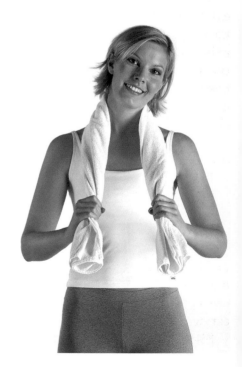

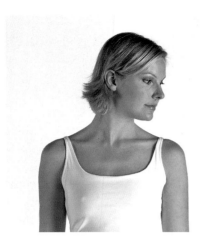
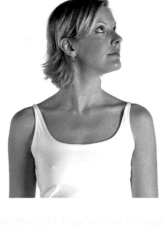
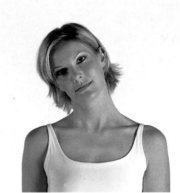
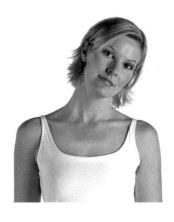

time without the help of a towel. Your head should be in the central position looking forward. Imagine a line, or axis, extending from the tip of your nose. Rotate your head on this axis, with your ear approaching the shoulder on each side. The nose should remain stable, moving neither up or down nor side to side.

■ TIP:

These simple and effective exercises help to reduce strain on the cervical spine.

There is a stabilizing and mobilizing component to all movement. The following exercises will help keep your cervical spine stable.

Sit down and clasp your

hands over the nape of your neck, as shown. Point your elbows forward at shoulder level so that your forearms touch. Rest your chin between your forearms. Pull forward with your hands while pushing backward with the nape of your neck. Keep your elbows at shoulder level and look directly ahead throughout the exercise. This will straighten your cervical spine. Maintain the muscular tension for a few seconds. Next, push your chin toward your elbows.

Never exercise the skeletal muscles of your spine without contracting the supporting muscles to stabilize it. This is especially important in the area of the cervical spine. The following exercises demonstrate which muscles to contract.

Place one hand on the side of your head and push. Create resistance by pressing your head against your hand in the opposite direction. Build up and hold the tension. Repeat on the other side and then with your forehead.

Not only mobilization...

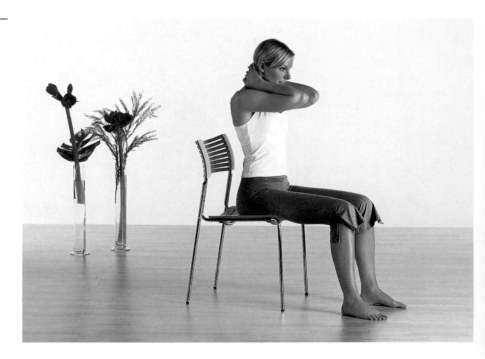

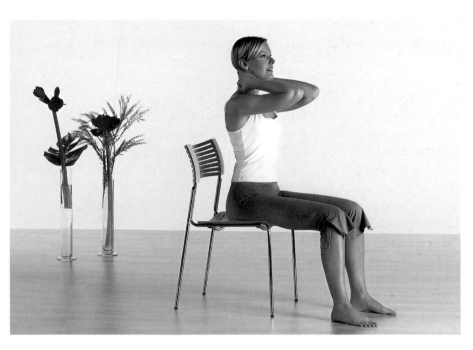

...but also
stabilization!

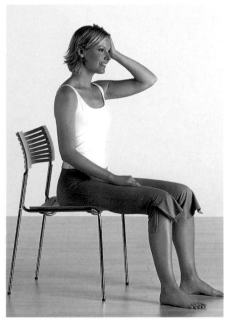

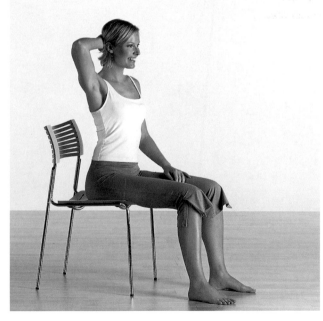

Other Ways to Exercise While Seated

After sitting for long periods of time, muscular tension decreases. As a result, many people end up in a slumped position. If that happens, you should either stand up and move around or perform a few exercises to regain muscular tension.

This first exercise is particularly useful for straightening the thoracic spine: Put your hands on your chair next to your buttocks. Focus your eyes on a spot directly in front of you throughout the exercise. Hold the edges of your chair and bend your elbows slightly. Next, hold your upper body taut by pushing your palms against the chair and extending your elbows. Stretch your neck as if trying to touch your head to the ceiling. This helps straighten your cervical spine.

Active rest while sitting

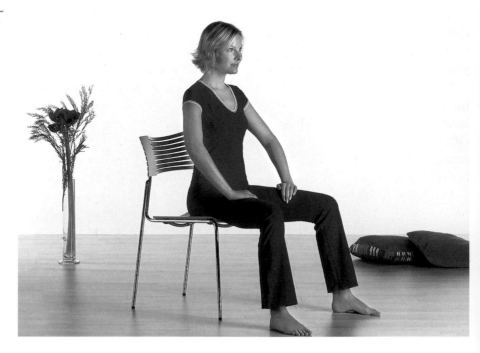

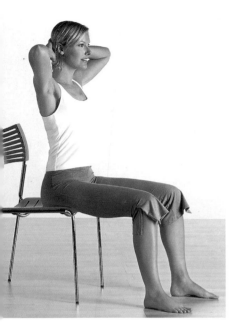

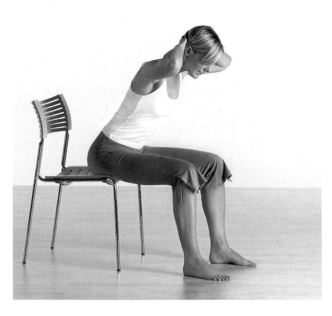

You can time the rhythm of this exercise to your breath: Flex when you inhale and release your breath slowly as you exhale.

If you want to increase the intensity of the muscular contraction, do so gradually. Otherwise you may experience cramps. Always make sure to breathe freely.

Clasp your hands behind your head. Slowly pull your elbows toward your back. This pushes your breastbone forward, straightening your thoracic spine and increasing the tension in your shoulder girdle. Make sure not to tilt your upper body

backward. You can increase the contraction of your muscles by drawing your shoulder blades toward your spine. This is another exercise you can do in sync with your breathing.

The following exercise will help you gain better control over your upper body and spine. Breathe freely and keep your gaze focused in front of you throughout.

Clasp your hands behind your head. Draw your elbows toward your back, but this time bend your upper body forward slightly from the hip joints. (This is easier if you picture your upper

Controlling the straightened spine

body as a single unit.) Then draw your elbows toward your back to increase the tension.

Very specific stabilization of the shoulder girdle can be attained by performing different hand and arm movements. Raise both arms to shoulder level while you sit firmly. Bend your elbows at right angles, with your palms turned outward and your fingertips pointing forward. Contract your muscles by pulling your upper arms and elbows slightly backward. Keep them at shoulder level. At the same time, draw your shoulder blades in toward your spine and push outward with your hands. Imagine that you are pushing against a doorframe. Do not straighten your elbows. If it is difficult for you to contract your muscles, try this exercise without your hands. Make sure your upper arms and elbows do not drop below shoulder level.

Now hold out your arms and

Exert force against imaginary resistance.

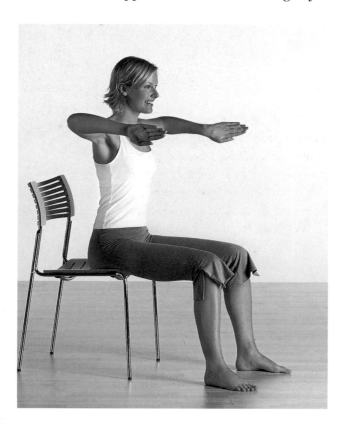
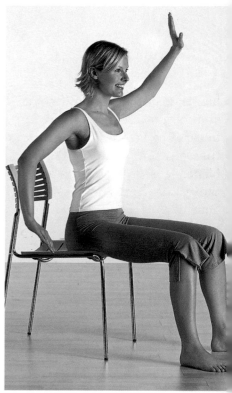

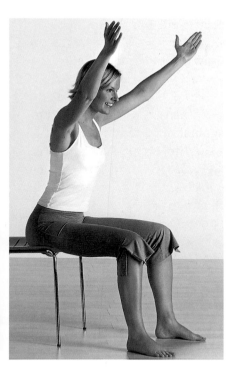

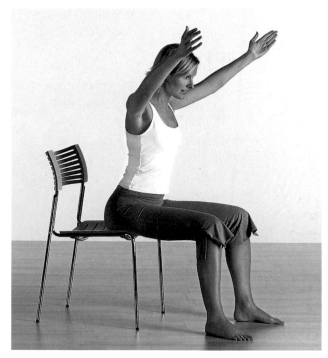

A variation

hands diagonally, as in the photo on the right. Contract your muscles as before. It is important that you pull your shoulder blades toward your spine and that your palms push outward. Your upper body should remain in the starting position throughout.

The next exercise targets a variety of muscle groups.

Imagine that you are stretching a large rubber band between your hands. Keeping your elbows slightly bent, extend your arms and raise them to form a big V with your fingertips pointing at the ceiling. Your upper arms should be alongside your head. Draw your shoulder blades in toward your spine while pushing your arms as far up as possible. Your upper arms should be further back now, near your ears. Your upper body and spine should remain in the starting position.

■ **TIP:**

Repeat these simple exercises throughout the day to reduce strain on your cervical spine.

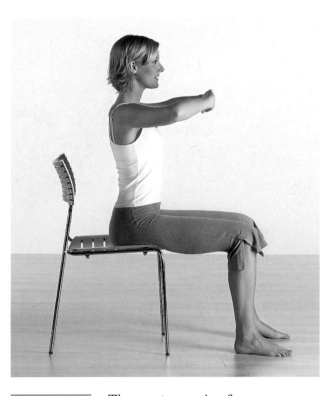
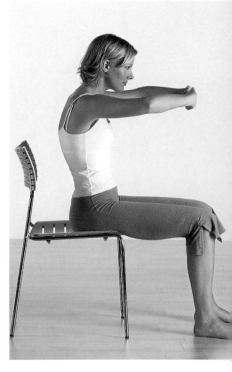

Stabilizing the shoulder girdle

The next exercise for your shoulder girdle requires a different arm position. Raise your arms to shoulder level with your elbows slightly bent. Point your palms outward as if you were pushing something away. Draw your shoulder blades in toward your spine without lowering your arms. Then push your shoulders straight forward. This slightly arches your thoracic spine. Your arms should remain at shoulder level with your elbows gently bent. This stabilizing exercise straightens your entire spine.

How to Help the Spinal Column While Standing

As humans developed from the tetrapod to the biped state, our rib cage and shoulder girdle adapted to functional changes. We no longer use them for forward movement; instead they have supporting and sustaining functions. However, your arms reach their functional potential only if the shoulder girdle is sufficiently stabilized.

Many people, even those who are young, have a limited ability to straighten their spine. This phenomenon is a prime example of muscular imbalance and is caused by chronically relaxed muscles and underdeveloped stabilizing muscles. The following stretching exercise targets a group of muscles that, if underdeveloped, accentuate disorders of the thoracic spine.

Stand sideways next to a wall with your feet apart. Rest your hand and forearm against the wall, with your elbow approximately at shoulder level. Stretch by turning your entire upper body away from the wall without moving your shoulders. Make sure your spine is stable.

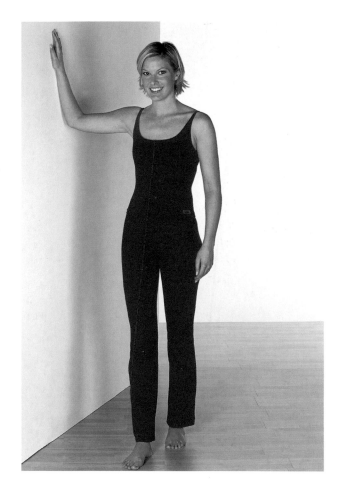

Stretching your pectorals

Be sure not to arch your back. Repeat on the other side.

The next exercise stretches the large pectoral muscles. The pectoral muscle, one of the powerful muscles that control your arm, originates in the chest. It puts a lot of tension on the shoulder joint because it connects your upper arm to

The stabilizing muscles of the spine must be in balance.

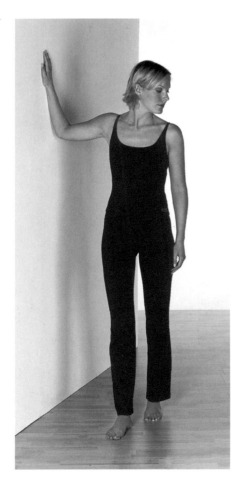

your torso. Make sure to stretch it very carefully in order to avoid straining the shoulder joint. This is especially important if your shoulder girdle is unstable.

The pectoral muscle is shaped like a fan. If viewed from the perspective of your rib cage, the individual muscle fibers converge toward your upper arm. Stretch this muscle by resting your hand and forearm against the wall somewhat above shoulder level. Repeat this exercise regularly.

The following exercise requires you to execute a sequence of movements not commonly performed. Stand straight and face the wall. Put your hands against the wall so that your elbows are slightly bent. Spread your legs and look directly ahead, between your hands. Push your thoracic spine backward and arch your back, keeping your elbows bent. Slowly lower your upper body toward the wall. Try not to bend your elbows any further as you approach the wall. Your shoulder blades will then move inward toward the spine.

Be careful not to arch your back. Increase muscular

tension. Your shoulders will now move forward and your shoulder blades will move away from the spine.

This exercise targets the serratus anterior muscles, which are located on the side of your chest and connect the ribs to the shoulder blade. Their primary function is to enable the forward and backward "sawing" motion of the shoulder area.

Do not perform this exercise by simply bending and straightening your arms. You must stay focused during this exercise, which requires you to move in

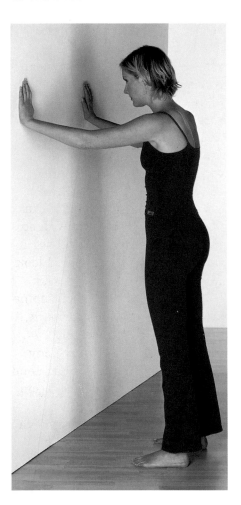

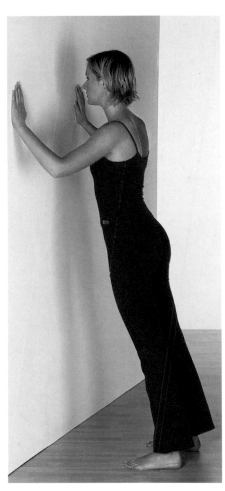

Stabilizing your shoulder blades

Controlling pelvis position

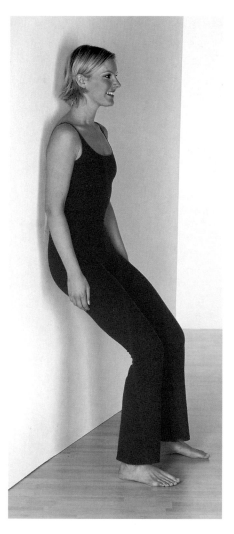

points of your body, you will discover what is good for your spine and pelvis. The interplay between the tilting and straightening of the pelvis should serve as a reminder of the spinal structure's dependence on the position of the pelvis.

This exercise makes you aware of the way your pelvis moves. Stand about a foot from the wall with your feet hip-width apart, then lean your torso against the wall. Keeping your gluteus and shoulders in contact with the wall, begin to tilt your pelvis away from it. If you feel that you are not doing this correctly, try pushing out your abdomen, making it round. In the final position, your pelvis should be tilted sharply and your lumbar spine stretched to a degree that exceeds its natural curve. This "spiral" position is called swayback, which is generally considered faulty posture. Next contract the abdominal and gluteal muscles and rotate your pelvis backward until your lower back is flat against the wall. If you are flexible, your lower back may now be completely flat against the wall. Do not hold your

unaccustomed ways. Keep your elbows bent while performing it.

There are many opportunities to work on your posture as you go through your day. A wall can be very useful as a support surface. By learning the contact breath during muscular contraction.

In the next exercise you will build up even more muscular tension.

Stand slightly away from the wall with your feet spread hip-width. Distribute your weight evenly between both legs. Relax your arms and let them hang. Lean your thoracic spine and shoulder girdle against the wall. Contract your muscles by placing both of your palms on the wall and pushing. Keep your arms straight. Your contracting abdominal and gluteal muscles will straighten the pelvis and push your lumbar spine against the wall. Be sure to keep your shoulders on the wall throughout the contraction.

When you build up and relax muscular tension, do it slowly and consciously. You may want to time your breathing with the exercises: Exhale when you straighten your pelvis and inhale when you start to relax. This helps you to continue breathing freely.

For the next exercise, stand about half a step away from the wall with your feet again spread hip-width. Lean your back against the wall and bend your knees at right angles. You will definitely feel the tension in your leg muscles, and this can make it difficult to move your pelvis. At first, just switch between tilting and straightening your pelvis while holding the position.

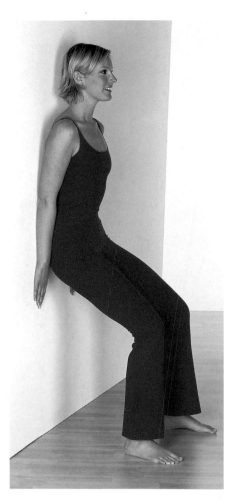

Simultaneous contraction of abdominal and back muscles

Once you can do this without difficulty, intensify the muscular contraction as follows: Hold your arms up with your elbows bent and the backs of your hands and arms resting on the wall, as shown on page 55. Lean your head back. When you straighten your pelvis, push your shoulders, your arms, and finally your hands against the wall.

Now lift your arms above shoulder level to rotate your shoulders outward. This straightens your thoracic spine.

Variation of active pelvis control

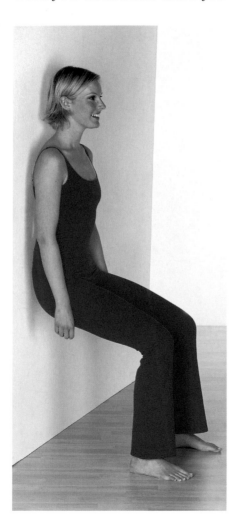
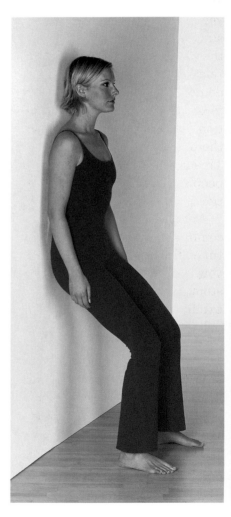

Keep your pelvis stable so that the movement of your arms does not affect the position of your spine.

Do not use so much force that the lower part of your back remains against the wall. Relax the muscles in your arms and shoulders when you start to tilt your pelvis. After some practice, start to time your breathing to the rhythm of contraction and relaxation. Make sure that you do not hold your breath. Failing to breathe during the contraction of the torso muscles raises the pressure in the rib cage. This can be problematic for people who suffer from circulation problems.

Another variation is to combine moving your pelvis in time with your breathing. Tilt your pelvis. This will relax your stomach muscles while you exhale and straighten your pelvis as you inhale.

■ TIP:

The combination of pelvis movements with conscious breathing draws one's body awareness to the lower spine.

You can also exercise stabilizing muscles without leaning against a wall by simply

contracting them. Do this while sitting in the office or standing in line.

For the next exercise, stand

Additional use of the shoulder muscles

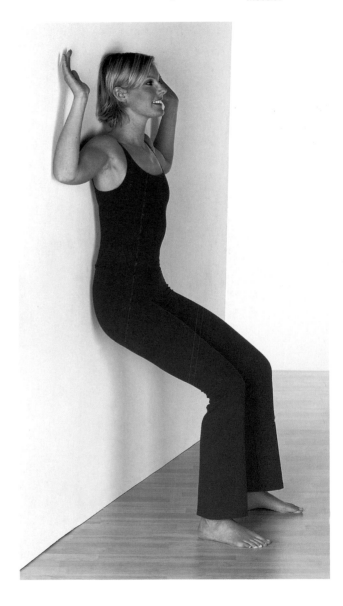

Stabilization in an upright position

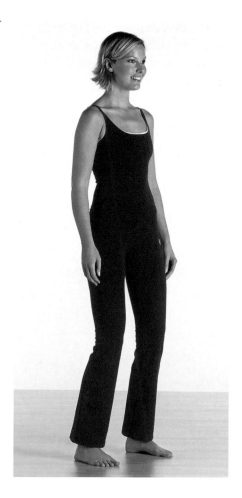 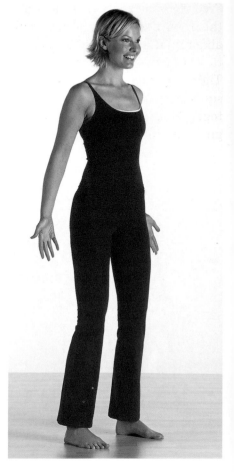

straight with your feet hip-width apart. Bend your knees slightly. Distribute your weight evenly between both legs. Relax your arms and let them hang. Contract the muscles by turning your hands and arms outward so that your thumbs point away from your body.

Continue turning your arms until your palms point outward. Rotating your shoulder joints in this way straightens the thoracic spine. Further enhance the effect by slightly raising your rib cage and stretching your neck as if trying to touch your head to the ceiling. Do not arch your back. You can prevent this by actively contracting your abdominal and gluteal muscles to stabilize your lumbar spine. Tighten your gluteal muscles by squeezing your buttocks together. Make your shoulder girdle more stable by drawing your shoulder blades toward your spine. Keep your knees slightly bent throughout the exercise.

If you have difficulty stabilizing your shoulder girdle, you can try the following, simpler alternative to the exercise (see

A variation

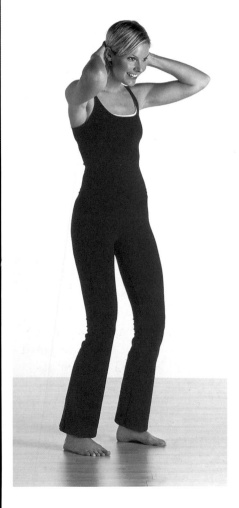
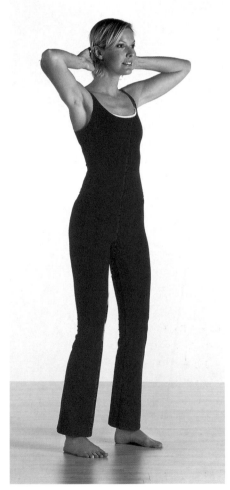

pictures on page 57). Bend your knees slightly with your feet spread hip-width. Clasp your hands behind your head with your elbows pointing forward. Slowly pull them toward your spine. The contraction of your stomach muscles controls the position of your pelvis. Finally, draw your shoulder blades in toward your spine.

Conscious contraction of abdominal and trunk muscles

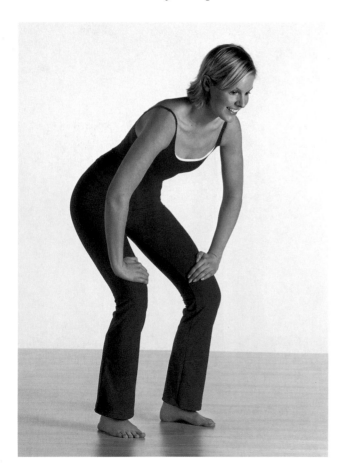

■ **Contracting muscles without the support of a wall takes practice.**

Although this book includes exercises for all components of the musculoskeletal system, here we are focusing on the muscles of the shoulder girdle. Increase muscular tension in your trunk and stomach as follows: Stand upright with your feet spread hip-width. Bend your knees until you can touch your thighs with gently bent elbows. Your hands should rest slightly above your knees and your fingertips should point inward, toward each other.

Start the contraction by pushing your hands against your thighs. Arch your back slightly to activate your stomach muscles. Straighten your thoracic and cervical spine. Imagine that you are being pulled upward by a thread. Always breathe freely. You can exhale during contraction and inhale during relaxation, which will also establish a certain rhythm.

What's the Best Way to Bend and Lift?

Some of the most common daily movements include bending down to pick up objects. This movement puts increased strain on the spine. The reason for this is that the upper body is functioning as a long lever, as shown in the picture on the left. This especially affects the lumbar spine. The strain put on the spine in this position increases rapidly in proportion to the weight that you lift.

When you bend over like this, the pressure on the intervertebral disks is uneven.

Bending with straight legs puts strain on the spine.

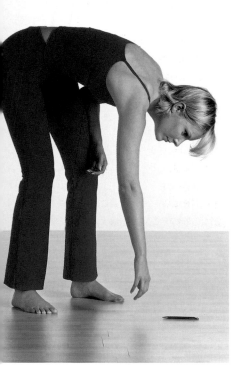

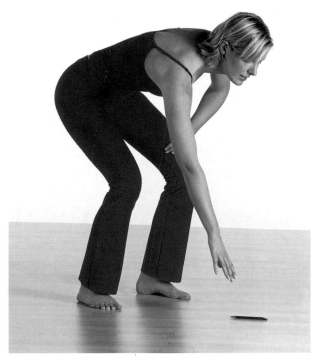

This puts a lot of strain on the intervertebral disks. When picking up small objects, try to bend down as shown in the right-hand picture on page 59. Support your upper body with your forearm by resting your hand on your leg. You can further decrease strain on the lower section of your back by bending your knees. When you lift heavier objects, try to keep your arms close to your body to minimize strain on your spine. This is easier when you bend your knees. Most of the strength you need to lift an object is provided by your leg muscles. If you keep your legs straight, your back muscles do all the lifting. Lifting becomes easier still when you spread your legs and position yourself as close as possible to the object you want to lift. Remember to breathe freely, especially when you lift and carry things. If you cannot keep up a smooth breathing pattern while you are lifting, inhale when you feel strain on your spine. You may want to practice bending down and lifting a few times with an empty box.

A short lifting distance helps protect your spine.

Another reason that bending down to lift things is such a problem for many is that a lot of people with back problems also have weak knee joints. Just like any other joint problem, this weakens the surrounding muscles. If you have weak knees, you should not try to relieve your back by using your leg muscles. Carry small objects only and divide up larger loads.

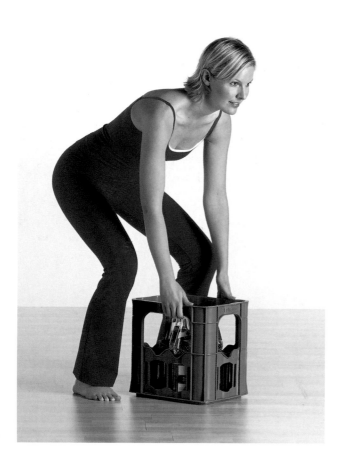

A Strong Back in the Morning

Not everyone enjoys the idea of exercising in the morning. However, many people exercise without even knowing it when they stretch upon waking. You should make this a habit and incorporate other stretching and contraction exercises into your morning routine.

Again, you do not have to do every single exercise in this book. Finding which ones work best for you will increase the likelihood that you will do them regularly.

Start your day by stretching in all directions and contracting different groups of muscles. Make fists while extending your arms, or stretch your toes and feet while straightening your legs. Try to time this to the rhythm of your breathing. Inhale slowly and deeply while you relax and let the air escape while you stretch. Do not hold your breath while you stretch. It may negatively affect your blood pressure.

Stabilize your pelvis and torso as follows: Lie on your back with your legs and upper body in a straight line. Grab one knee with both hands and

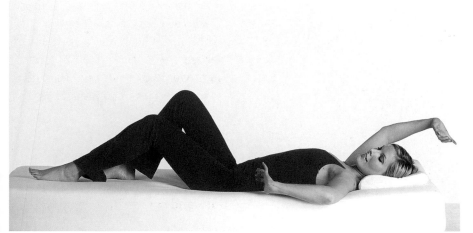

Stretching "wakes" your muscles.

pull your thigh in close to your chest. Firmly flex the toes of the straightened leg toward you, pushing your heel in the opposite direction. Keep your other leg close to your upper body throughout the contraction.

■ **TIP:**

Muscular contraction stimulates not only your muscles but also the cerebrum. Exercising really helps you wake up.

Simple and systematic contraction exercises in the morning...

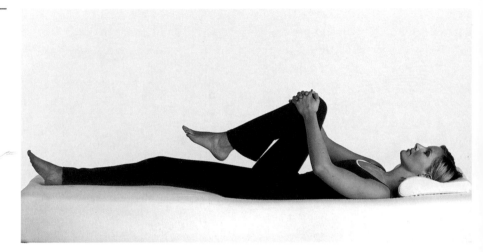

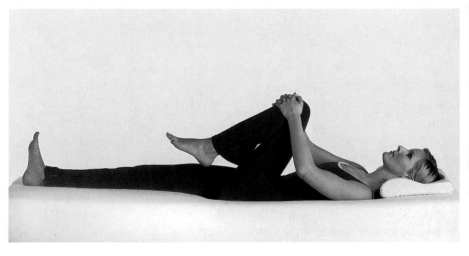

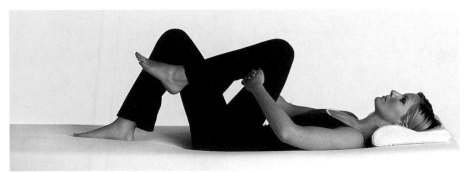

...are complemented by simple stretching exercises.

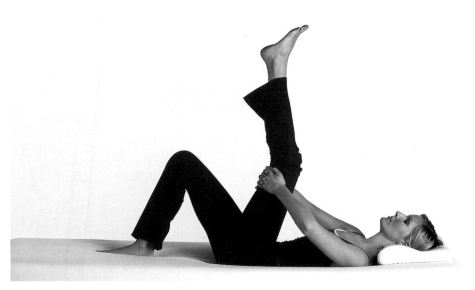

For the following stretching exercise, lie on your back and bend one leg. Clasp your hands behind the other leg and pull your thigh toward your chest while bending your knee. Slowly straighten your leg without changing the position of your thigh. Straighten your leg only as much as you comfortably can.

The bottom of your foot should now face the ceiling. Stretch your calf muscles even further by flexing the tips of your toes toward you (see photo on page 64).

For the next exercise lie on your side. It may help to lie at the edge of your mattress. One leg should be on top of the other

A Strong Back in the Morning

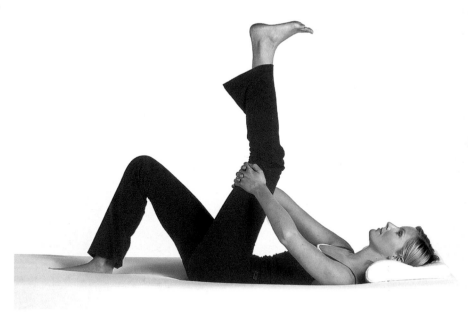

and both should be bent at right angles at the hips and knees, as shown in the top photo on page 65. Slowly turn your top shoulder toward your back and let your head follow. Your legs should remain in the starting position throughout the exercise. This is easier if you put the hand of your lower arm on your upper knee. If you can do this easily, you should move your upper arm back diagonally when you turn.

Change the effect of this exercise on your spine by bending your legs at different angles. If you keep them almost straight,

the rotation starts in your lumbar spine. If you bend them further, the rotation shifts to the upper sections of the spine. Intensify this stretch by keeping your lower leg straight in the starting position. Do this only if you are flexible and your spine rotates easily (see bottom picture on page 65). Repeat this exercise on the other side of your body.

Some people cannot perform these exercises without experiencing pain. *Stop immediately if you experience pain or discomfort during this exercise.*

The next exercises focus on building up muscular tension.

In addition to the mobilizing positions, the body tension can also be increased. You may find it more comfortable to place a pillow under your abdomen instead of lying flat, as shown on pages 66–67.

Lying on your stomach, spread your legs hip-width apart and rest them on the inner edges of your feet. Rest your arms above your head with your elbows bent and your upper arms forming a right

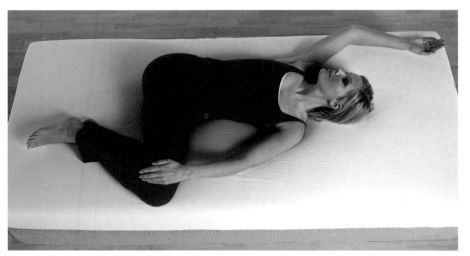

To perform this stretch, focus your attention on your spine.

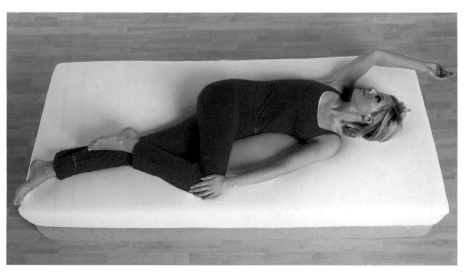

angle with your body, as in the photo on page 66. Keep your head facedown or turn it to the side. Build up muscular tension by pressing the inner edges of your feet against the mattress while keeping your legs straight. Squeeze your buttocks together to further increase muscular tension.

Raise your head and look down. Your forehead should be a couple of inches above the mattress. Straighten your thoracic spine even further by drawing your head away from your spine. Imagine that you are being pulled lengthwise by a thread.

The following exercise involves the muscles of the shoulder girdle and the torso: Build up muscular tension as before, then lift your arms an inch or so and hold them parallel to the mattress. Then draw your shoulder blades in toward your spine. Hold your head so that you're looking down at the mattress. Make sure you continue to breathe freely as you increase the tension.

If this exercise is too difficult at first, try this variation: Start in the same position as before, with your hands next to your face, but turn your arms inward. This will force you to raise your head somewhat; be sure to keep your thoracic spine straight as you do so. (Alternately, you can keep your arms by your side and stretch your fingertips toward your feet, as shown in the bottom picture on page 67.) You should now be able to draw your shoulder blades in toward your spine.

Increase your body tension.

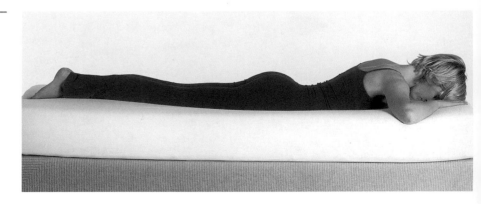

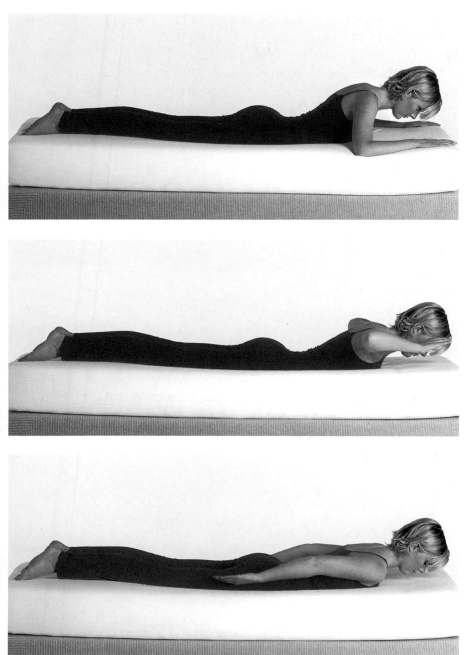

The abdominal muscles do not perform solely support and motor functions. When they contract, they increase the pressure in the cavity of your stomach, which helps stabilize the lumbar spine. The following exercise shows how to contract the muscles of your torso and stomach.

Lying on your back, bend your legs and grab your knees from behind, as shown. Your thighs should be pulled toward your upper body. Use your hands to bring your legs even closer to your chest as you start to exhale. Raise your head and look at your knees. Release your grip and relax the tension while inhaling deeply. Focus on keeping the rhythm of your breathing in sync with the muscular movement.

The next exercise leads to a stronger contraction of the

With the help of abdominal contractions the lumbar spine can be stabilized immediately.

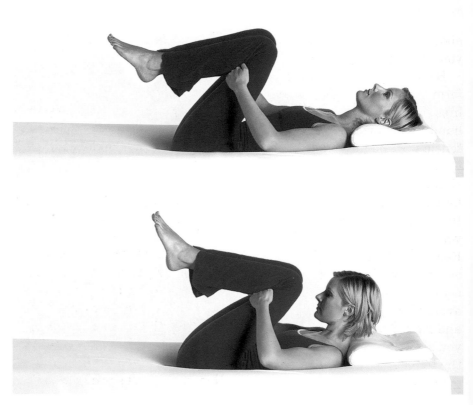

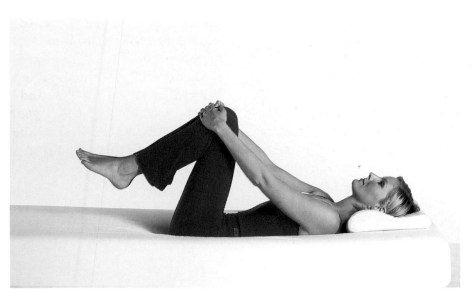

abdominal muscles. Make sure you breathe freely throughout it.

Bend your legs so that they form a right angle with your hips. Hold your knees with both hands, as shown. Build up tension by pushing your knees against your hands, while simultaneously using your hands to pull them toward you. Imagine that you are pushing your knees toward the ceiling. Keep your head straight in order to avoid straining the cervical spine. (You can also avoid this by raising your head and looking at your thighs when you start the contraction.) Relax the tension as you finish exhaling.

This exercise is fairly difficult for beginners.

■ TIP:

Avoid pressure breathing by combining contractions with exhalation. This helps you to continually breathe freely.

The following exercises will create stronger muscular tension in your abdomen and torso.

The abdominal muscles consist of straight and oblique, or diagonal, muscle fibers, which connect the upper body to the pelvis. These muscles can flex and turn the torso, straighten the pelvis, or do both at the same time. Their support function is to stabilize the torso against the pelvis and vice versa.

Bend both legs while lying on your back. Your knees should be directly above your hips and your lower legs should be parallel to the mattress. Your head can rest on the mattress or you may want to support it with a flat pillow.

Put your hands next to your buttocks with your arms outstretched and your palms facing upward. The position of your arms will cause your shoulder joints to turn outward. This outward rotation makes it easier to straighten your

thoracic spine. Keep it straightened throughout the entire exercise.

Slowly lift your head as you start to exhale and look at your knees. Continue to turn your hands and arms outward while simultaneously pushing them toward your feet. Consciously intensify the muscular tension around your shoulders while drawing them toward your spine. Return to the starting position as you finish exhaling.

Lie on your back again and raise your legs. Point them upward so that your hip joints form a right angle.

Additional contractions for your abdominals

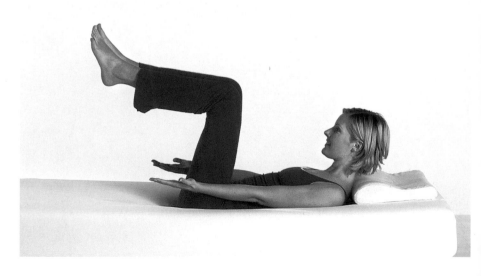

Try to straighten your legs as much as possible. Place your hands alongside your buttocks, with your palms facing upward. Push your legs upward, while pressing the backs of your hands against the mattress. It is easier to perform this exercise if you bend your hips even further. Make sure that you continue to breathe freely throughout. Relax a little afterward. Use your pillow to support your upper back. Spread your legs hip-width and straighten them. Bend your elbows so that they form a right angle with your upper body.

Your hands should be above your head, as in the photo on page 72.

Individuals who suffer from a lack of mobility in the shoulders may find this position uncomfortable. If so, simply avoid this exercise entirely.

Supporting your upper body with a pillow makes it easier both to straighten the thoracic spine and to breathe. Do not mistake this position for an arched back position, however. An arched back puts strain on the lumbar region of the spine.

Pay attention to your breathing for a couple of

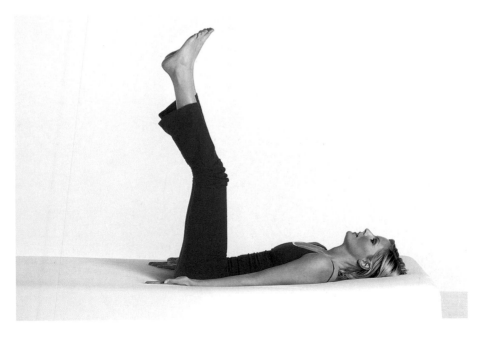

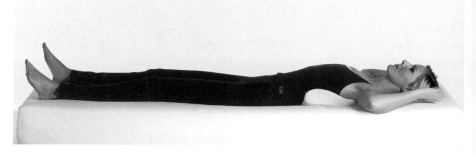

minutes. Try consciously to trace the length of your breathing intervals. Note the activity of your rib cage and stomach. Then try to direct the flow of your breath into your abdomen as you inhale, imagining that you are becoming wider and rounder. Then exhale slowly.

This exercise does not focus on deep breathing and taking in the right amount of air, but it does help you breathe in a relaxed way. If you have difficulty directing air to your abdomen, place your hands on your stomach as you inhale. Concentrate on your stomach movements. Take a couple of minutes to observe your breathing but do not relax too much. Remember that you are exercising to be more active when your start your day.

When Getting Up Is a Problem

People who suffer from back pain know how difficult it can be to straighten their torso and stand up from a horizontal position. The following exercise shows how to get up without pain by supporting your entire upper body. It will not only help

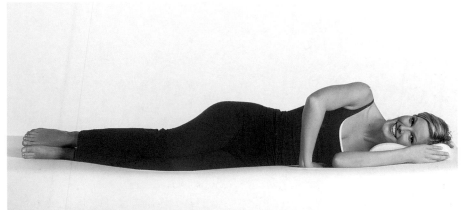

Protect your spine while getting up from the lying position.

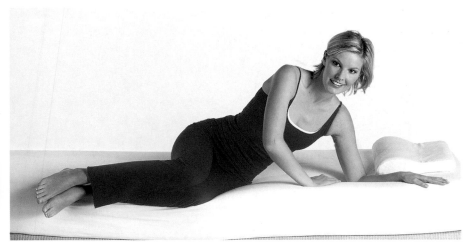

Rotate to sit up, maintaining your body tension.

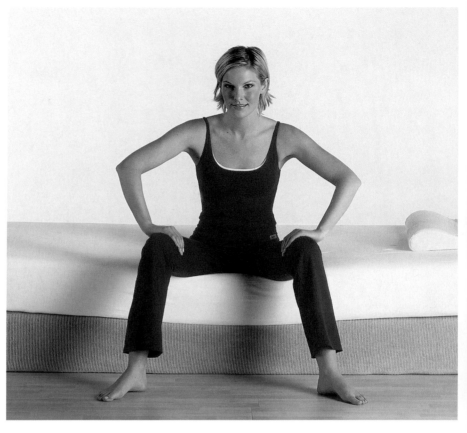

people who already suffer from back pain but also prevent future spinal damage.

Bend one leg first, then the other, while lying on your back. Turn sideways so that you are close to the edge of your bed. Your legs should form right angles with your hip and knee joints. Rest your head on one hand for support and place the other in front of your chest. Lift your upper body as you push down on the bottom arm and supporting hand. At the same time, push your legs forward and turn them until your feet reach the ground. Maintain the muscular tension of your entire body until you are in a sitting position. Now sit and relax for a moment.

Maintain this muscular tension as you stand up. Put

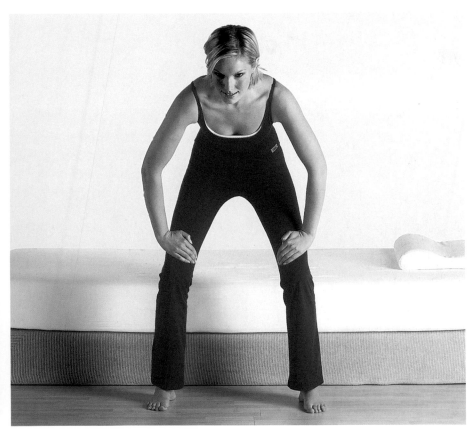

...and while getting up

both palms on your thighs, slightly above the knees. Bend your elbows. Tilt your upper body forward until your center of gravity is over your feet. Straighten your legs. Support yourself with your hands until you feel that your body is in balance. Make sure that your spine is stable during the entire movement. Breathe freely throughout. Stand up by straightening your hip joints.

A Stable Back After Getting Up

Having started your daily routine with a couple of exercises in bed, the bathroom is your next opportunity to fit in a few more. Here it may be possible to work different groups of muscles that help stabilize your posture. Remember that you always need to focus while doing these exercises. You will

Assume a relaxed starting position to actively correct your posture.

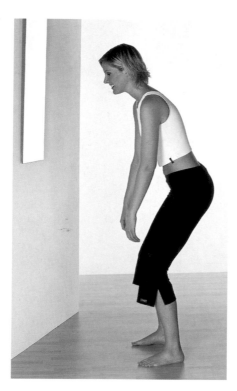

not achieve the required muscular tension or perform the movements correctly if you do not. The exercise descriptions in this book are merely a guide for certain positions and movements; you must actively follow the guide to discover which exercises actually improve your physical condition. Regularly perform those that appeal to you and let them influence your habits of posture and movement.

After getting up, your first activity is probably to bathe. It is common, when you arise, to slump in front of the sink, brushing your teeth. Just like you, your musculoskeletal system is not quite awake yet. The muscle groups responsible for supporting the upper body are not in use. This lack of stability puts more strain on the skeletal system.

Correct your posture as follows in order to activate the potential of your muscles: Set your feet apart slightly wider than your hips, distributing your weight evenly between both legs. Bend your knees while slightly tilting your upper body forward. Relax your arms and let them hang at your sides. Your fingers should point to the ground and your back should be slightly curved.

Now straighten your upper body by stretching the individual vertebrae. Start with your thoracic spine and end by raising your head so that you are looking directly into the mirror. Your knees should be slightly bent throughout and you should feel some tension in your thighs. When you tilt your upper body forward while washing your face or brushing your teeth, make sure to support your torso in order to decrease strain on your spine. You can do this by resting your forearm on the edge of the sink. Remember to keep your knees bent to minimize the strain on your spine.

Another way to do this is to bend your knees and rest one hand on your thigh, which stabilizes your upper body.

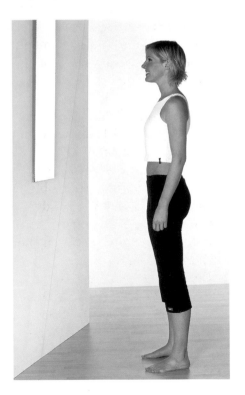
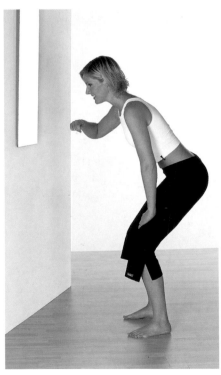

Left: Be aware of your postural habits.

Right: Even small changes in your habits of movement can reduce the strain on your spinal column.

Other Activities for a Healthy Back

While sitting

Many of us spend the majority of the workday sitting in front of a computer. To alleviate the strain on your lower back, try the following relaxation and stability exercises.

Sit in your chair and spread your legs. Now lower your upper body until it rests on your thighs, keeping your spine stable. Relax your arms and head. Close your eyes if you want to. Focus on the rhythm of your breathing to see when you are inhaling and when you are exhaling. Make sure to breathe freely.

Take a couple of deep breaths and straighten your spine again while exhaling. Start with the lumbar spine and continue with your thoracic spine. Finally, straighten your cervical spine.

Take a passive
sitting break...

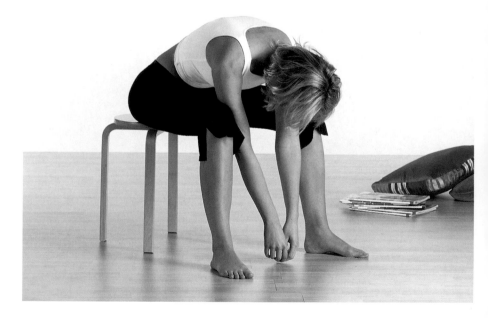

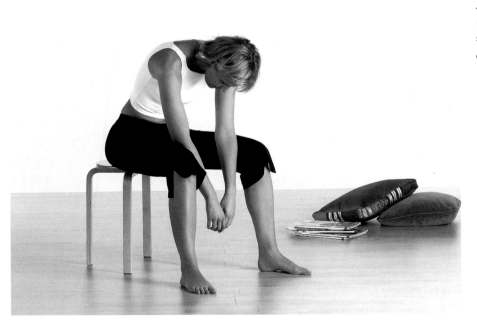

...then actively straighten up afterward.

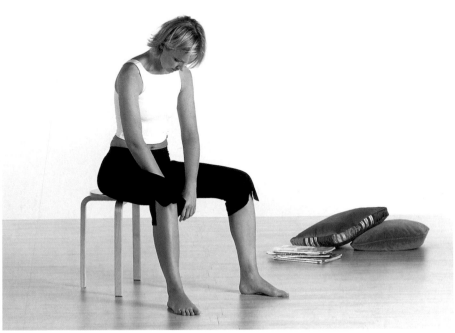

Do not sit up completely. Keep your upper body bent slightly forward and tilt your pelvis forward as well. Raise your rib cage. Make sure your head is centered between your shoulders and look directly in front of you. Proceed by doing some stretches.

Some people have problems breathing freely when they bend forward in this fashion. If this is the case, do not do it. Try the following exercise instead: Sit upright in a stable position and start to relax. Arch your back. Rest your forearms on your thighs, then close your eyes.

Always contract your muscles after relaxing in your seat.

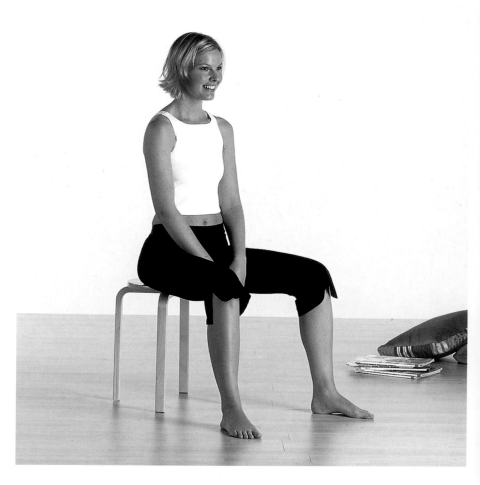

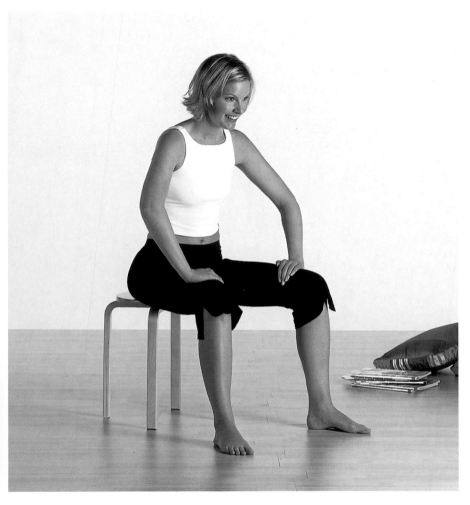

Deep abdominal breathing can be relaxing.

Concentrate on the rhythm of your breathing. Focus on inhaling, then on exhaling. Slightly contract your abdominal muscles. Imagine that you get wider and rounder as you inhale.

Do not resume your working position abruptly. After a relaxation break you should give your body some time to prepare for sitting upright again. Open your eyes and sit up slowly. Take a couple of deep breaths and stretch thoroughly.

The combination of muscular tension and breathing can help you wake up.

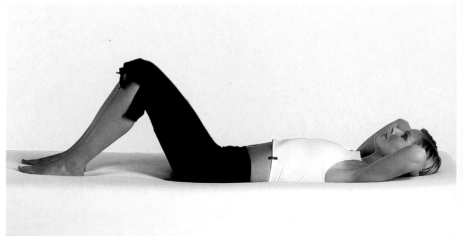

While reclining

The following exercise will wake you up in seconds. It is a combination exercise that comprises muscular contraction, relaxation, and rhythmic breathing.

Lie faceup with your hands clasped behind your head. Bend your knees and put your feet flat on the mattress, as shown. Focus on the rhythm of your breathing until you can clearly distinguish inhaling from exhaling. Push your elbows down slightly when you inhale and relax as you start to exhale. Once you have coordinated the flexing and relaxing of your muscles with the rhythm of your breathing, you can intensify the contractions. Continue to breathe evenly. Never hold your breath.

Once you can do this seamlessly, lift your lumbar spine off the mattress slightly while inhaling. Let it sink back down as you exhale. This causes you to breathe very deeply. Now lift both your lumbar region and rib cage off the mattress. Lower your body and relax. The following exercise also combines muscular contraction and relaxation with rhythmic breathing.

The pressure exerted by your feet straightens your pelvis and flattens your lumbar spine. Your abdominal muscles contract as well. You can lift your pelvis even further by increasing the tension of your stomach. This

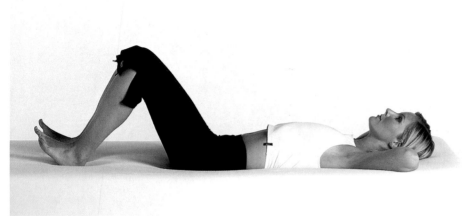

Building up muscular tension

straightens your upper body until your thighs are aligned with it. Following these steps in reverse order, return to the starting position. Do not relax your stomach muscles until you are sitting up.

Do not hold your breath. It is common to hold your breath while you contract your muscles, especially in people who do not exercise regularly. Doing each exercise very slowly will help you avoid this.

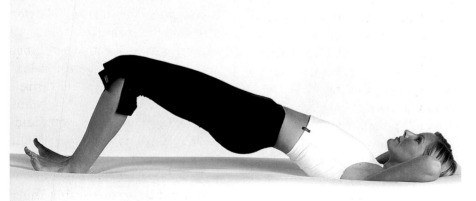

Increasing muscular tension

Once you are able to build up muscular tension and move your pelvis in a smooth rhythm, you can start to focus on your breathing. Concentrate on inhaling first. Begin contracting the muscles as you start to inhale. Do not lift your buttocks at this point. Relax while you exhale.

Increase the intensity of muscle contraction by raising your pelvis when you inhale and lowering it when you exhale. Once you are more familiar with this exercise, you can further intensify the muscle contraction as you wish.

It may be difficult to breathe deeply throughout this exercise because you are contracting your abdominal muscles and your body therefore directs the air into your rib cage. Pay attention to the movements of your rib cage while you perform the exercise. When you inhale, you activate the muscles between your ribs, which in turn raises the entire rib cage.

Try the following to straighten your thoracic spine: Lie on your back with a cushion for support. Bend your legs and spread them hip-width, as shown. Rest your arms above your head and bend your elbows.

You should control the tension of your abdominal muscles so that you continue to breathe freely.

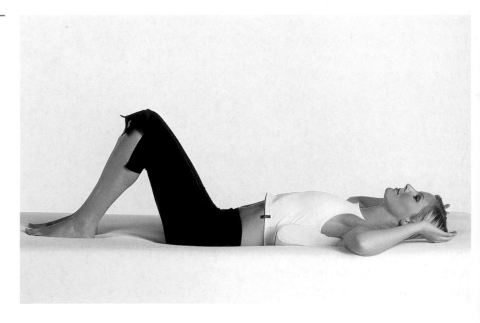

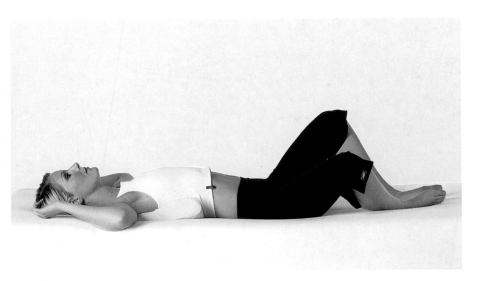

Now lower your knees toward the mattress. Focus on your breathing, then relax. This exercise demands that you straighten your thoracic spine because you are supporting your shoulder with a cushion. The movement of your arms helps straighten the thoracic spine.

Many people develop disorders in the shoulder joints early in life, which diminishes their flexibility and may make it impossible for them to move their arms in the way this exercise requires. If you suffer from such a disorder, try to exercise the affected body part with a more muscle-specific workout plan. However, if you have problems performing common movements or are in chronic pain, see a physician.

The next exercise rotates the spine. Lie on your back with a pillow supporting your upper torso. Rest your arms next to your head with your elbows at right angles, as shown in the top photo on page 86. Place your feet flat on the mattress.

If you can do so comfortably, move both legs down on the same side, making sure that your shoulders remain on the mattress. Stay in this position for a few moments, breathing deeply. Then bring your legs to the other side.

The next exercise targets your stomach muscles and

A variation

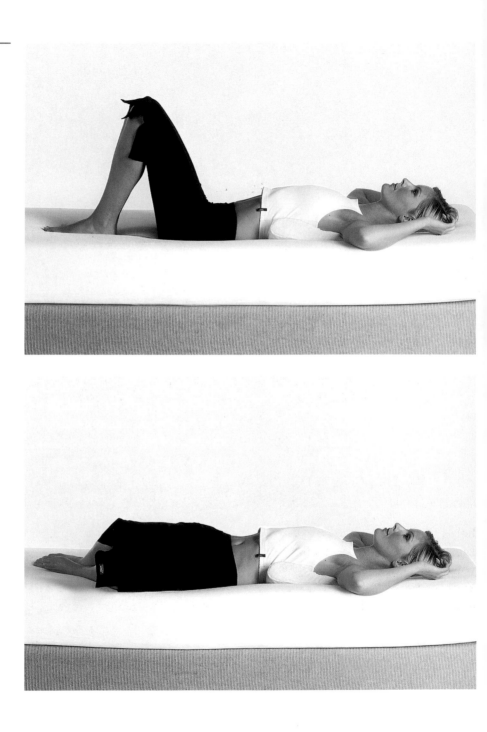

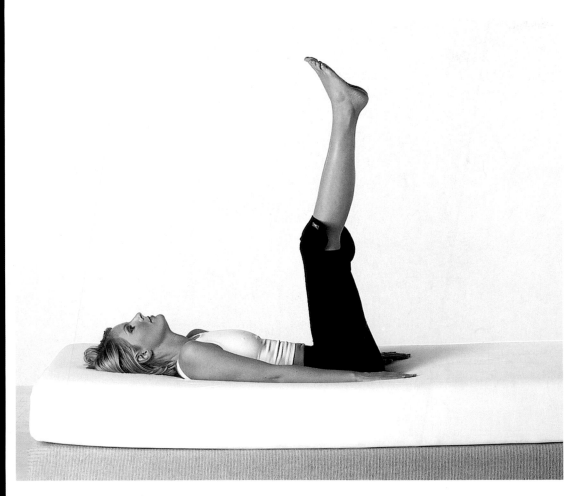

helps you straighten your pelvis. Lie on your back and stretch your legs toward the ceiling. Your legs should form a right angle at the hip. Place your palms down alongside to your buttocks. Push your feet upward and press down against the mattress with your hands. This lifts your pelvis an inch or so.

Intense
abdominal
contraction

You should practice a combination of breathing and muscular contraction.

While standing

Breathing is an unconscious function. You need not pay attention to it, but you can change its rhythm by focusing

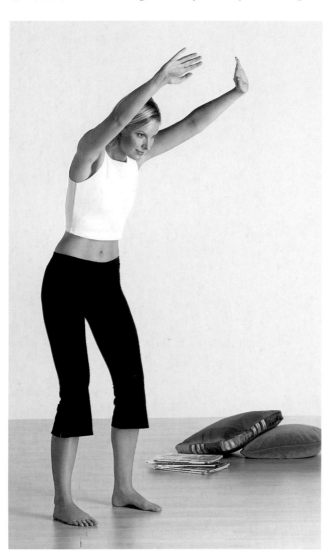

on it. Learn to distinguish between the volume of your breath, which is how much air you inhale, and the way you breathe, for example, into your stomach or into your chest.

Taking a deep breath is fairly easy; it is much more difficult to switch from breathing into your chest to breathing into your stomach, which is called abdominal respiration.

Timing the rhythm of your breathing to targeted muscular activity may be difficult for those unaccustomed to working out. When you exercise, it is important that you contract and relax your muscles gently. The first time you perform an exercise, do it without focusing on your breathing. Never interrupt the flow of your breathing or hold your breath. You will find that combining your breathing rhythm with timed muscular contraction has a stimulating and refreshing effect on both your body and your brain.

Stand with your feet hip-width apart and your weight evenly distributed between your legs. Raise your arms so they are parallel to the ground, and lower your upper body slightly. Do not shift your weight forward or backward.

Bend your knees gently and look between your feet. Now arch your back and push outward with your hands. Contract your abdominal muscles. Imagine you are drawing your navel toward the center of your body.

Do not raise your upper body as you proceed. Lower your hands to your buttocks with your fingertips pointing toward your body and your palms facing backward. Keep your knees bent and straighten your head. Push your hands away from your body. You should now be looking diagonally at the ground. This muscular contraction straightens your spine. Once you become familiar with this exercise, you can focus on your breathing.

Start to breathe more deeply as you build up muscular tension. Do not exhale too suddenly or for too long. Exhale as you arch your back and push your hands forward. The contraction of your stomach muscles helps you exhale. Slowly change your position when you start to inhale again. Increase the muscular tension while you continue to inhale.

■ TIP:
Paying attention to your breathing may conflict with contracting your muscles. Practice them separately.

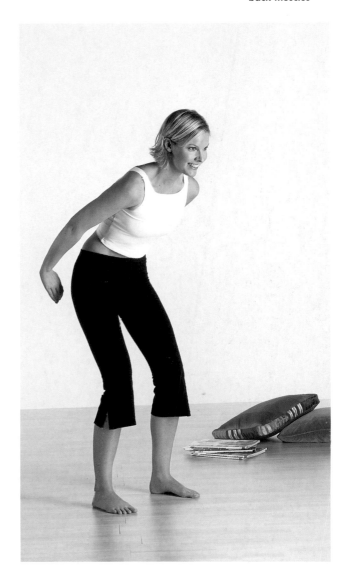

Contracting your back muscles

Try to inhale into your stomach cavity by relaxing your abdominal muscles. This activates your back extensors. However, if these muscles are unable to sufficiently stabilize your upper body or if you have other difficulties, for example because you are overweight, try the following alternative.

Stand up straight with your knees slightly bent. Spread your

Left: Contract your back muscles

Right: Arch your back as you exhale.

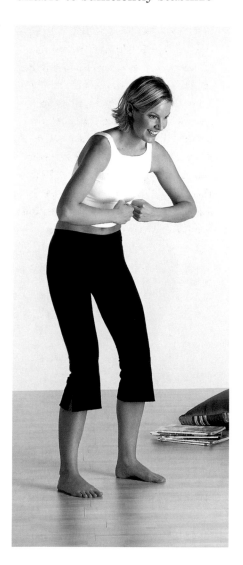
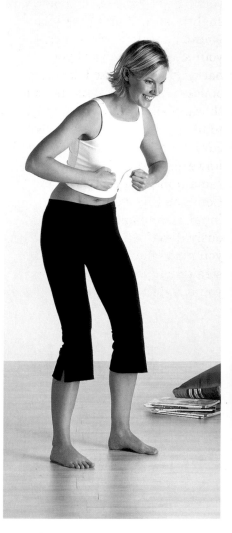

legs hip-width apart. Clench your fists and put your hands next to each other in front of your navel, as shown in the far-left photo (p. 90). Bend your upper body forward until your shoulders are directly above your knees. Your back should be slightly arched and your elbows pointed outward. Next, draw your shoulders toward your back, as in the near-left photo opposite. This straightens your thoracic spine and brings your lumbar region into its natural curved position. Push your head upward. Your feet and legs remain in the same position. Combine this exercise with inhaling and exhaling as previously described. Inhale while you arch your back, and straighten your spine while you exhale.

■ **TIP:**

In the preceding instructions your breathing should be harmonized with regulated movement and muscle contractions. With practice you should be able to do this exercise easily. Once you have learned to listen to your body, the effect is broader. Breathing is one of our bodily functions that we normally do not take notice of, but it is something that we can influence. The interaction of breathing, contraction, and movement can be multifaceted. One of the fundamental suggestions of this book is that you pay attention to your breathing during the exercises. This is a further opportunity to get in touch with your body by experiencing it in a new way.

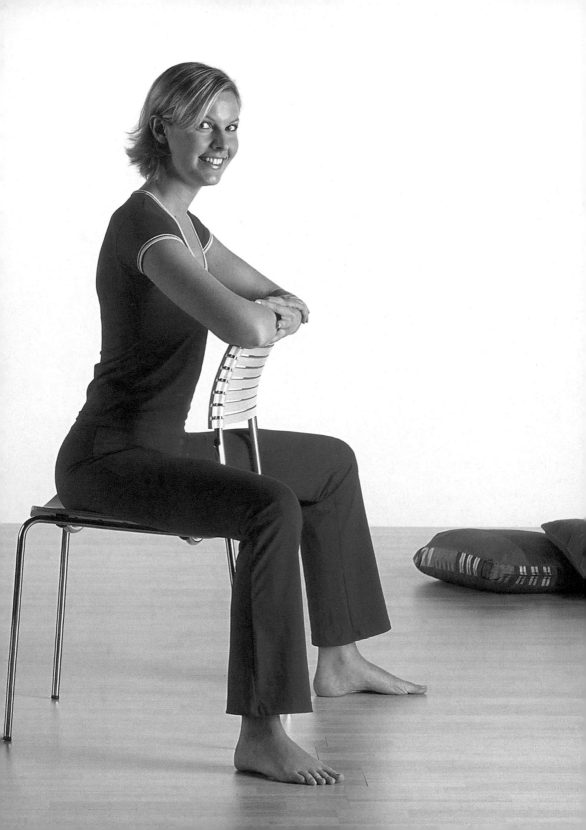

Index

About the Author

Helmut Reichardt was born in Germany in 1953 and began studying high school education at the Technical University of Darmstadt, outside Frankfurt. After becoming a physical therapist, he resumed his studies at the University of Tübingen, near Stuttgart. At the same time, he was certified as a sports physiotherapist. He received a masters degree in athletic pedagogy and sports biology in 1985. Until 1989 he was a member of a research team at the Institute of Athletic Research at the University of Tübingen.

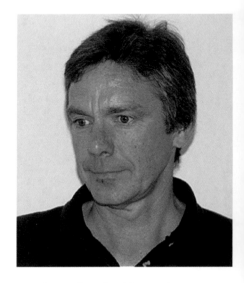

Mr. Reichardt has been a physiotherapeutic coach for young athletes since 1981 (German National Track and Field Association, German National Volleyball League, German Basketball Association). In 1989 he became an independent adviser for athletic and health concerns. In this context, he has been actively involved in projects for the Bavarian Association for Continuing Adult Health Education in Schools. He also has many years of experience in educating coaches for this program.

Mr. Reichardt has been running his own physiotherapeutic practice, including a center for physical therapy, since 1989. After relocating his practice, he is now working with two partners in rehabilitation and injury-prevention research.